Complex PTSD

10 Holistic Steps to Tame Triggers, Outshine Anxiety, Transcend Trauma, and Live Your Best Life

C.W. Lockhart, PhD

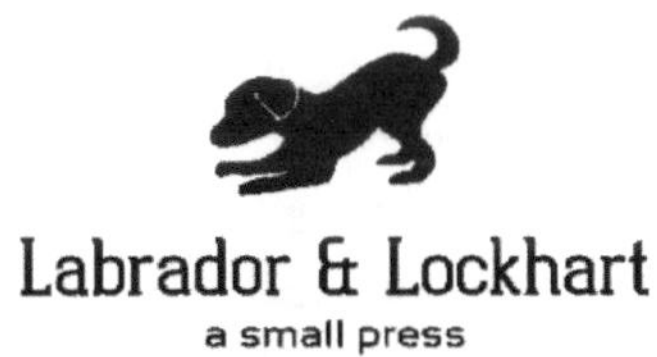

Labrador & Lockhart
a small press

Publisher's Note

This publication is meant to provide reliable and well-researched information regarding complex PTSD. Publication is sold with the knowledge and awareness that the publisher nor its affiliates practice or offer psychological services. This publication is not intended to replace professional services.

 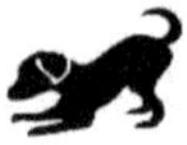

Published in the United States by Labrador & Lockhart Press, LLC
Ocean Shores, WA

LabradorandLockhart.com

Lockhart, C.W.,1967 – author.

Complex PTSD: 10 Holistic Steps to Identify Triggers, Manage Symptoms, Reduce Anxiety, and Live Your Best Life / C.W. Lockhart, PhD

Trade Paperback ISBN-13: 979-8-9909091-1-3
Hardcover ISBN 979-8-3289380-4-4
(Labrador & Lockhart Press, LLC)
ISBN-10: 8990909106

First Edition

~For Garret and Dessie

And for my little Brothers and Sisters-in-arms.

For those who served with me, and for those who came before.

I will always hold a space for you in my heart.

I will stand here, right next to you, in solidarity.

Please remember, you are never alone.

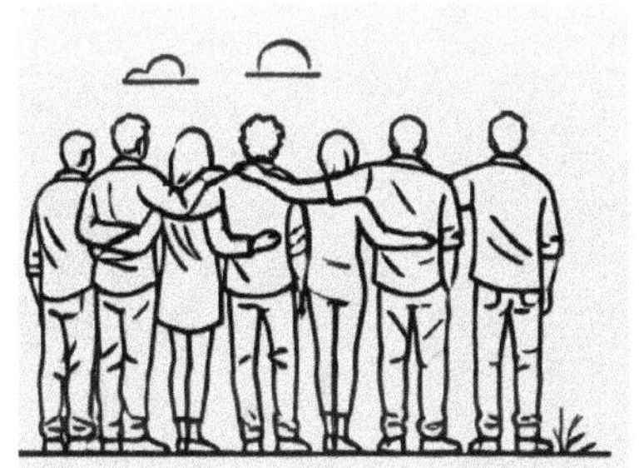

CONTENTS

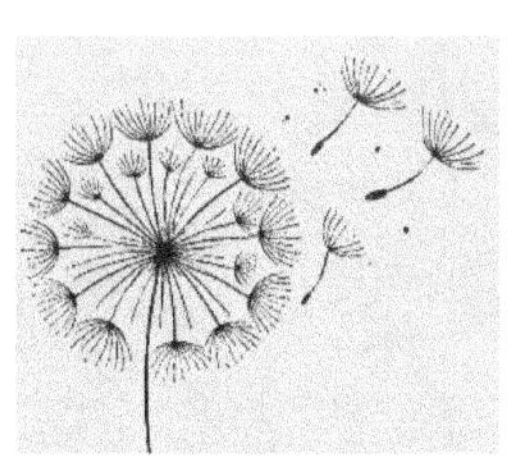

Complex PTSD

10 Holistic Steps to Tame Triggers, Outshine Anxiety, Transcend Trauma, and Live Your Best Life

Step 1: Decide to Move Forward

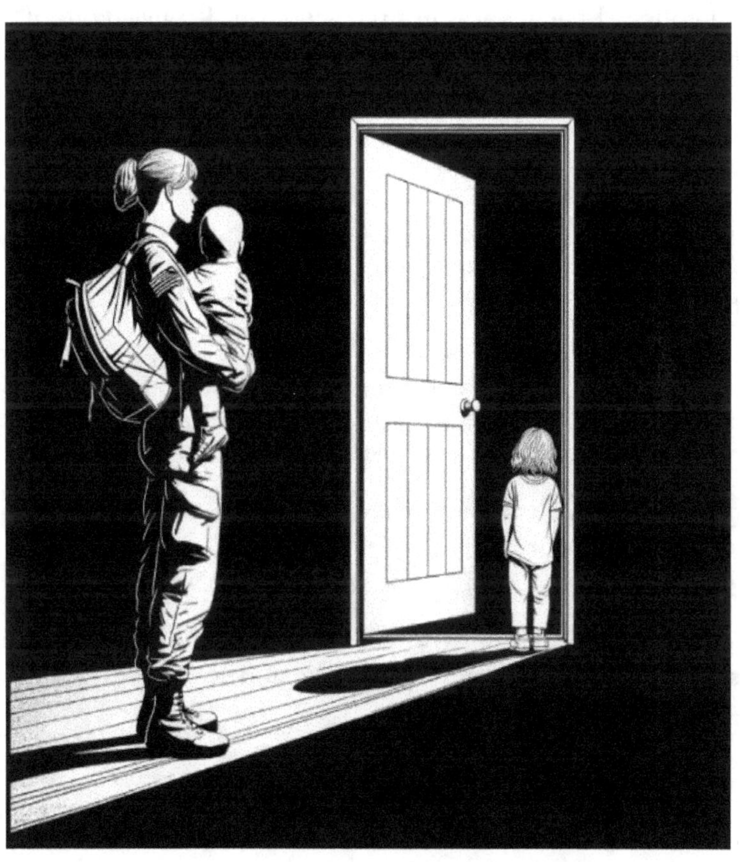

That first night was difficult. The wind wailed through the towering pines surrounding my new home. A naked branch reached out to scratch against my bedroom window, and a wayward pinecone skittered down the tin roof.

I bolted upright in bed, my heart racing as I tried to soothe myself. "Calm down, Girl," I whispered. "You know it's just the wind."

Of course, I knew it was just the wind. But I crawled out of bed anyway, tossed on my fluffy bathrobe, and pattered downstairs to ensure the doors and windows were locked. Once satisfied, I climbed back upstairs and sought refuge beneath a sea of blankets.

"Now, quit being a scaredy-cat," I scolded myself. "Go back to sleep."

Sleep didn't come easily that night. Nor did it come on most nights to follow. Bleary-eyed, I haunted the small rooms of my two-story cabin, revisiting the front and back doors and checking all the window latches.

I made the rounds twice that night, just to be sure. But as time marched on, so did my hypervigilance. My nightly security routine grew into three, four, and sometimes seven rotations per evening.

At first, I chalked up my odd behavior to stress. Newly divorced, a first-time homeowner, and a single mom to three little boys, how could I be anything *but* stressed?

Oh, and let's not forget about work. I was in the Army, serving my second tour on recruiting duty. It was a rotten job made exponentially worse by a supervisor with a lewd mouth and inappropriate intentions.

Of course, it wasn't just the divorce. Nor was it the responsibility of home ownership or single parenting. It wasn't even my total jerk of a boss.

"You've been through way worse," I reasoned. And that was the absolute truth. But something was different. Something inside me had cracked. As the tiny fissure widened, I found myself leaking a mixture of fear, grief, and rage. I just couldn't keep my head together anymore. And it made no sense to me at all.

One morning, I stood in the hallway, fully dressed in crisp camouflage and mirror-shined black combat boots. The eldest had already caught the school bus, successfully starting off our day. The other two needed to be dropped off at daycare before I could make the morning commute.

With the baby on my hip and a toddler at my feet, I was ready to go. All I had to do was turn the doorknob. But I just couldn't.

Overnight, the front door had turned into the darkest of passageways, a portal into a hostile world so chaotic and foreign. I did the only logical thing I could think of: I called in sick. Next, I put a movie on for the kids, undressed, slipped back into my fluffy bathrobe, and made myself a double Bloody Mary.

This phenomenon repeated itself regularly, as did my responses to it. Sometimes, it predictably followed a difficult night. But other times, it occurred rather unexpectedly, like after a great weekend with pals or a restful sleep or when I thought I was feeling fantastic.

Little by little, I was losing my place in the outside world. Everything I had once taken for granted now seemed unattainable, dangerous, and overwhelming. The charming cedar-planked walls of my little cabin in the woods, which was supposed to be my sanctuary, had become a prison instead.

These episodic moments of despair weren't isolated events on just a few bad days. No. These moments were the culmination of years of trauma, both psychological and physical. For years, I had neatly boxed up and filed away these unpleasantries somewhere in the dark recesses of my mind. But the boxes were popping open faster than I could smack them down.

I had always been a tough girl, farm-raised, athletic, and much stronger than I looked. In boot camp, after a rigorous session of hand-to-hand combat training, my drill sergeant shook his head in disbelief. "Soldier," he said. "You hard! You harder than a woodpecker's lips."

I'd often repeat the drill sergeant's funny compliment. I used it as an affirmation of sorts. *Damn right, I'm hard. Harder than a woodpecker's lips.*

Unfortunately, quirky affirmations, my overreliance on humor, and misplaced bravado left me ill-equipped to fight in the war against *Complex PTSD*. Drowning it all in vodka wasn't working either. I needed new strategies, and I needed them fast.

My journey through trauma wasn't a new thing brought on by an Army enlistment. Trauma rations were not issued items, like extra gear in my olive-drab duffle bag. No. The injuries began in early childhood and stretched into my teens and throughout my years of military service.

Each year of military service added another layer and a heavier burden to bear. I tried shielding myself from the pain with temporary fixes. Often, these fixes worked—until they didn't.

At a ridiculously low point, I self-referred to a military mental health clinic. I was seeking assistance with alcohol abuse and sleep deprivation. A young officer, wearing gold bars newer than my boots, conducted the intake interview.

"Are you homicidal?" he asked.

"No, Sir." I shook my head.

"Suicidal?"

"No, Sir."

"Wanna go A.W.O.L?"

"No. Not really, Sir."

"Well, then." He paused, putting down his pen and pushing up his wire-framed glasses.

I swallowed the growing lump in my throat and fought back threatening tears.

He stood, signaled me to do the same, and said, "Drive on, Soldier. Drive on!"

That was it—end of the intake interview. I had been dismissed.

In the prescriptive wisdom of the young lieutenant, I was simply ordered to *drive on.* Drive on? What in the hell does that even mean?

During the road trip from *Madigan Army Medical Hospital* to my recruiting station in Longview, Washington, I contemplated *driving on.*

I could *drive on* right into a tree or *drive on* into oncoming lanes of traffic.

I could even *drive on* right through the bridge railing and down to the swift green river below.

Thankfully, contemplations of suicide were fleeting. By the time I made it back home, rage had replaced despair. I had not single-handedly put myself in such a mess. But it was clear. I was all on my own.

There was nothing to do about it but toughen up. So, I laced my boots tighter and stuffed my emotions down further. I cut back on the booze and picked up a hobby, soapmaking, which turned into a decent little side hustle.

Instead of drinking myself to sleep, I stirred batches and batches of creamy olive oil soap. Soap and soap-making supplies soon filled up my tiny kitchen. I stirred late into the night, almost every night, until I was too tired to hold the wooden spoon.

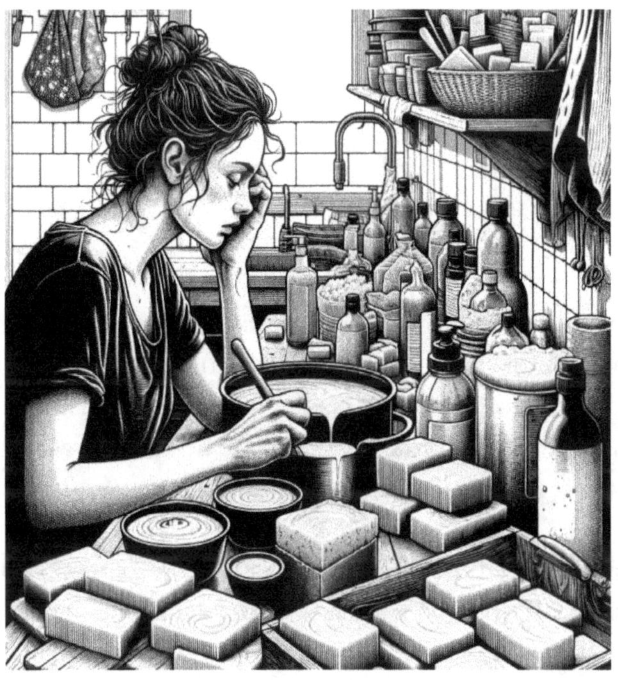

I wasn't sane. Nor was I completely sober. But the boys and I were squeaky clean.

I held out like this for the next fourteen years. I remarried and completed a master's degree and a PhD. I even left the Army to earn my commission in the Coast Guard.

From the outside, I was the epitome of a *hard charger*. I was a living, breathing poster child of all things related to *Driving On*.

My gosh! Wouldn't that young lieutenant from Army Mental Health have been so proud?

As long as I stayed insanely busy, I could continue *driving on*. As long as I never stopped to think, I could keep my head straight. And as long as I never stopped running, I could keep the boogeyman off my trail.

But then, one day, everything changed.

Out of the clear blue sky, I was hit by debilitating attacks of migraine headaches. Sure. From time to time, I suffered an unexplained headache. But searing pain, tunnel vision, and projectile vomiting? No. The migraine headache was shockingly foreign.

Vertigo followed the migraines. Depression followed vertigo. And then, Agoraphobia joined the party, making me too afraid to even leave the house.

After twenty-four years of military service, my health had declined to such a point that there was nothing to do but retire.

But the madness of it all did not stop with retirement. Nope. The downward spiral continued, isolating me even more from the life I longed to live.

I realized that, eventually, I was going to have to deal with my shit and finally confront my relationship with Complex PTSD.

Simply put, it was time to take charge, kick-ass, and recover. But where to start? Does this sound familiar?

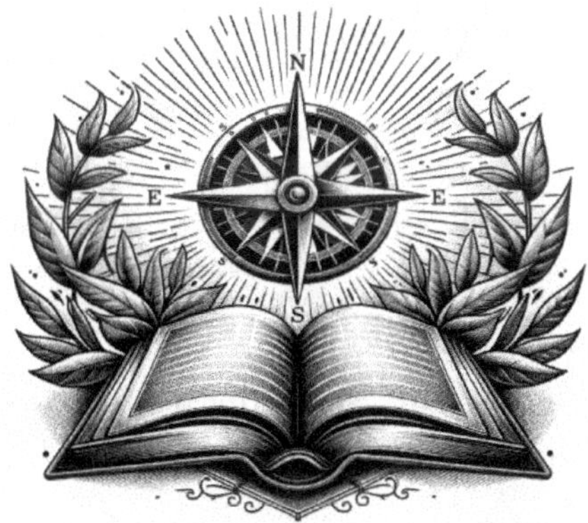

This book is born of necessity — a necessity to share integrative, holistic survival strategies.

These strategies continue to help me and have great potential to assist others, particularly veterans and, more specifically, women, regardless of military status, grappling with similar issues.

The purpose of this book is clear: to empower, educate, and inspire you to take charge, learn to tame triggers, outshine anxiety, transcend trauma, and live your very best life despite the challenges of Complex PTSD.

Throughout these pages, we will explore a variety of recovery modalities including art therapy, meditation, somatic therapy, therapeutic yoga, polyvagal theory, and nature therapy like camping and hiking.

We'll also explore some practical, everyday activities that stimulate connections between the right and left hemispheres of the brain. Interestingly, these activities share the same basic foundations of *Eye Movement Desensitization and Reprocessing,* or *EMDR.*

Wrapping it Up

Since those scary first nights in my little cabin in the woods, I have been successfully stumbling forward on my road to recovery.

While *I am* a doctor, I must note that I do not hold a license to practice medical or mental health. Instead, I hold a PhD.

My superpowers are analytical, critical, and creative thinking. And my weapons of choice are deep dives into research and self-experimentation.

Basically, I am my own guinea pig, and I'm so honored and grateful to share my findings with you.

This book interweaves personal anecdotes of resilience and recovery with actionable advice. I share my findings with sensitivity and support.

I will not share detailed accounts of personal trauma. You have your own burdens, and I shall not further weigh you down with mine.

At this point in my journey, *what happened* hardly matters. I acknowledge the past but choose to dwell in the present and embrace the future.

I write this as someone who has navigated the darkness of Complex PTSD and found a lit pathway through — and I believe you can, too.

You, the reader, whether a woman, military veteran, or someone who identifies with the struggles of Complex PTSD, are not alone.

This journey is for you. It's about finding strength in vulnerability and turning mere survival into a thriving and fulfilling existence.

Moving Forward

I invite you to join me with an open heart and mind. Are you ready to explore new and perhaps unconventional strategies that offer relief and illuminate the pathway you've been searching for?

Together, let's affirm that while our journeys through Complex PTSD are profoundly personal and undeniably challenging, these journeys are also brimming with opportunities for growth, recovery, solidarity, and victory.

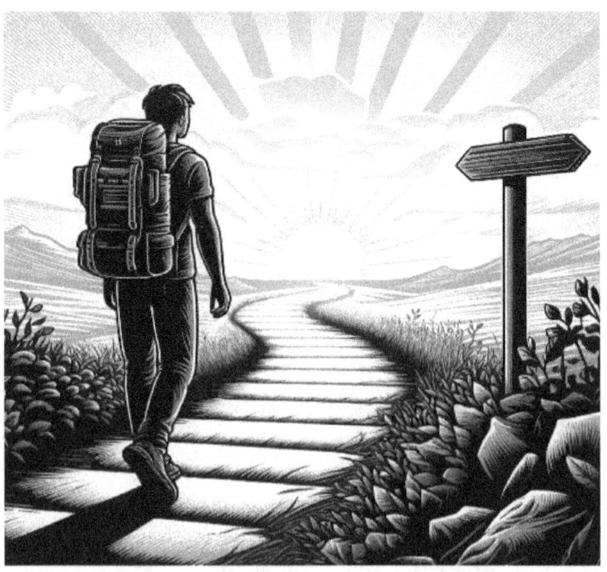

If you are still reading this book or listening to the audio version, I extend my heartfelt congratulations.

- ✓ **You've already accomplished Step 1: Decide to Move Forward.**

Let this little book be your guide to conquering Complex PTSD and reclaiming the vibrant life you deserve.

DISCLAIMER: *This book's holistic and integrative strategies are a collection of well-researched theories, practices, and personally lived experiences. This book is not a replacement for professional treatment. While these approaches may complement your current treatment path, I cannot guarantee these modalities will work for you. Afterall, there is no one-size-fits-all journey to recovery. We are all unique; therefore, I encourage you to discuss all activities with your care provider first.*

Step 2: Decode Complex PTSD

As you hold this book or listen to my voice in the audio version, perhaps you're feeling a mix of anticipation and apprehension.

The path to understanding complex PTSD is not just about identifying symptoms or mapping out therapies. The path is also about unraveling the complicated layers of your experiences and recognizing how deeply these experiences impact your sense of self.

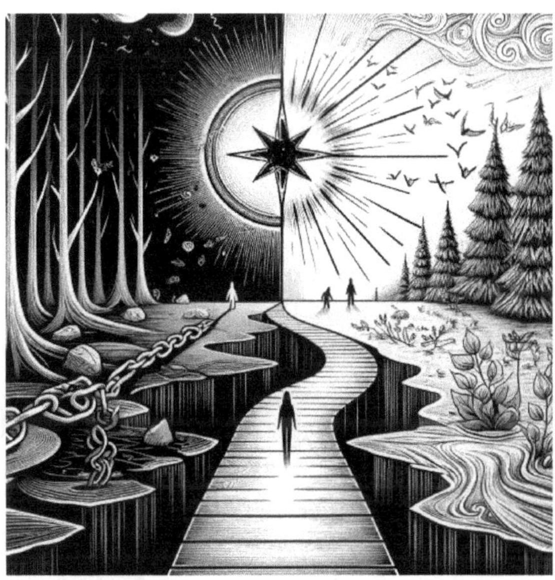

You might be wondering how your journey fits within the broader definitions of trauma and its aftermath.

This chapter serves as a foundation for scaffolding such knowledge, beginning with a clear differentiation between

Complex PTSD and *PTSD*, a distinction that is essential yet often overlooked.

Complex PTSD is not a straightforward diagnosis. It doesn't typically stem from a single event but instead evolves from a series of ongoing traumas or a prolonged traumatic experience, which can fundamentally alter your long-term emotional landscape.

This chapter will help you to recognize these subtle yet significant differences, providing a clearer lens through which to view your experiences and validate your feelings. Let's explore together.

With compassion and care, we'll examine the definitions, symptoms, and significant ways in which Complex PTSD can shape your life.

Complex PTSD vs. PTSD: Deciphering the Differences

When we consider the term *post-traumatic stress disorder* or *PTSD*, it is natural to visualize a soldier returning from war. For the most part, this makes logical sense.

- The *American Civil War* marked the diagnosis of *Soldier's Heart.*
- *WWI* introduced *Combat Fatigue.*
- *Shellshock* was popularized during WWII.
- Shellshock evolved into *Post-Vietnam Syndrome.*

Each new military conflict has pumped out a new term. In 1980, PTSD was officially established as an anxiety disorder. This has since been updated to a *trauma* and *stress-related* disorder.

With PTSD's historically significant military background, you may wonder if there is another term for non-combat-related PTSD. Again, this is a logical line of thought. But no. There is not a separate term.

Receiving that initial diagnosis of PTSD may often be very confusing, especially if you have always linked PTSD to combat-related terms, like battle-fatigue and shellshock.

I recall my own feelings upon hearing the original diagnosis. How can this be? This must be some mistake. Bewildered, I left my therapist's office in a state of denial.

I did what any academic worth her salt would do: I conducted my own research. It didn't take long. After the first round of journal articles, I accepted this simple truth:

- ✓ ***PTSD is the physical and mental manifestations of trauma brought on by exposure to dangerous situations or stimuli.***

How is C-PTSD Different from PTSD?

Complex PTSD, or C-PTSD, is a relatively new diagnosis. It was introduced in 1992 by Harvard psychiatrist Judith Lewis Herman. According to Herman, C-PTSD may occur after enduring severe stress over a prolonged period, often years.

This type of response to physical and emotional trauma may stem from a variety of sources.

Examples include, but are not limited to, the following:

- Long-term abuse during childhood
- Exposure to ongoing bullying
- Domestic violence
- Reoccurring acts of violence
- Participation in dangerous military operations
- Catastrophic natural disasters
- Sexual assault and ongoing harassment
- Prolonged situations where escape seems impossible.

The concept of PTSD, which is widely recognized and accepted, is that it can develop after a single traumatic event. On the other hand, C-PTSD encompasses not just the immediate reactions to distress. It also includes the ongoing impact on a person's entire self-belief system and how this person relates to the world.

Symptoms of C-PTSD may include the following:

- Difficulties regulating emotions, which may manifest as explosive anger.
- Persistent sadness without an identifiable source.
- Invasive thoughts and suicidal thoughts.
- Deep-seated betrayal with a distorted perception of the perpetrator.
- A preoccupation with seeking revenge.

Additionally, there is often a sense of hopelessness, a feeling that life will never get better, and these thoughts can pervade every moment of existence.

These symptoms are more persistent and broad ranging than those typically seen in PTSD, creating layers of complexity in both diagnosis and treatment.

C-PTSD & Self-Identity

Who are you? Not *what*, but *who*? The impact of complex trauma extends deep into the core of *who* you believe you are.

The chronic nature of this injury may disrupt your sense of identity and self-worth.

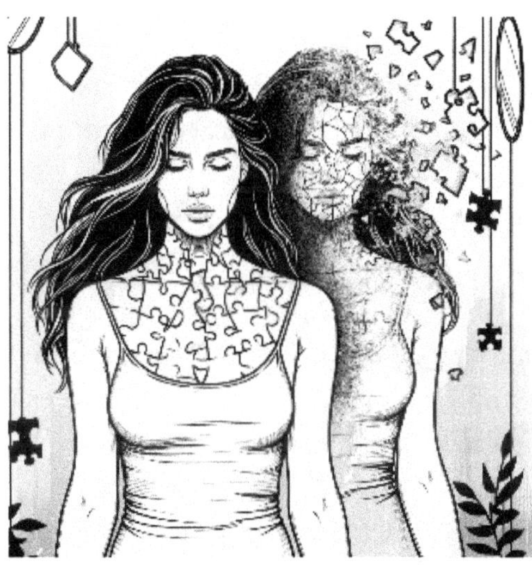

You may even experience a persistent sense of guilt or shame. You might somehow feel responsible for the trauma. You may even see yourself as severely flawed.

This erosion of self-concept is less about the symptoms of the trauma itself and more about *how* the ongoing abuse or living under the constant threat of danger distorts your view over time.

For me, ongoing exposure to trauma greatly impacted my concept of personal identity. For as long as I can remember, I have struggled with my sense of self. Growing up, I clung to the labels of tom-boy, jock, and class clown.

Later, I relied on my evolving military rank. I was Private, Specialist, Sergeant, Sergeant First-Class, and so on. I was my rank. And my rank was me. As long as I stayed in boots, I knew *what* I was but not necessarily *who* I was.

Recognition and Validation

Understanding and acknowledging the differences between Complex PTSD and PTSD is critical in the diagnosis process.

Recognition provides validation that what you are experiencing is *real* and that your feelings are legitimate.

It's not uncommon for individuals suffering from C-PTSD to have their symptoms misattributed, which may exacerbate feelings of isolation and misunderstanding.

For you, as someone who might be struggling with these complex emotions and memories, recognizing the depth and breadth of your experiences is the first step in taking charge of your recovery.

Give yourself permission to acknowledge the trauma. Acknowledge not just a series of events that *happened* to you but also recognize the deep influence trauma has on your concept of self and your approach to the world.

Personal Reflection Time

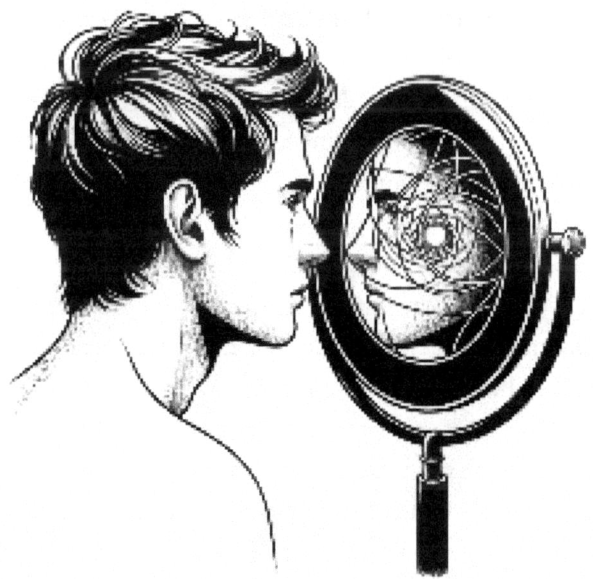

Developing a reflective practice will facilitate a deeper understanding and personalization of this information.

If you are in a safe space and feel ready to examine your history, I encourage you to reflect on the following questions. Feel free to journal your responses or simply ponder them in your mind.

Let's Start:

- How do my experiences of trauma fit into the definitions of C-PTSD that I have read about today?
- In what ways have I struggled with emotional regulation?
- How might my struggles with emotional regulation relate to my trauma history?
- Can I identify with the feelings of betrayal and hopelessness?
- Do I hold a distorted self-perception in my own life?
- How might recognizing and validating these experiences change how I view my recovery process?

Allow yourself time to digest, reflect, and revisit these questions. Connect the clinical information presented with your personal experiences. This will make the concepts more accessible and actionable.

If you currently receive care from a mental health practitioner, you might find it helpful to share these reflections during your next visit.

Your Brain on Trauma

Understanding how trauma rewires the brain is pivotal for anyone working to recover and reclaim their life. Without this essential knowledge, it's like wondering why a wound keeps bleeding without bothering to learn how to stop blood flow.

✓ ***A trauma wound is to the brain what a knife wound is to the flesh.***

Prolonged exposure to aggravating stimuli, as in chronic abuse or high-tempo military operations, may lead to significant changes in the brain's structure and function.

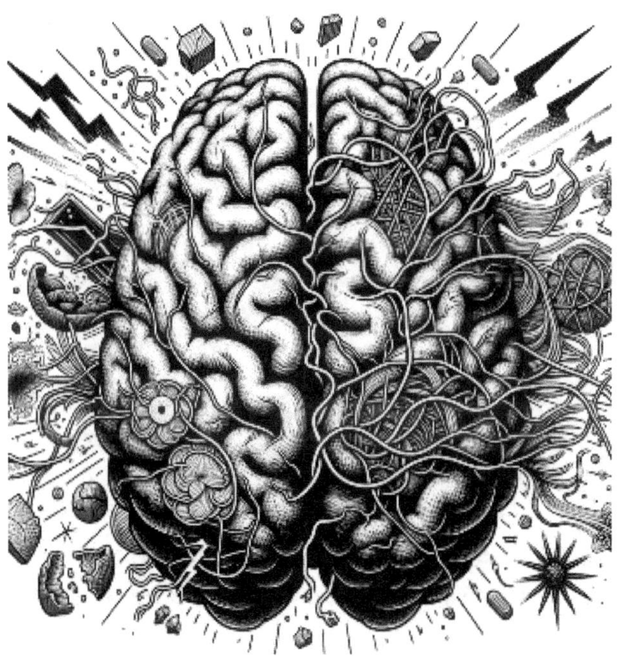

These alterations occur in the very areas that control our emotions, memory, and our sense of threat.

Fundamentally, this exposure reshapes how we perceive and interact with stimuli from the world around us.

The Hippocampus:

While our beautiful brains are stunningly adaptable, they are also incredibly sensitive to prolonged stress.

Trauma can shrink the *hippocampus*, the part of the brain involved in learning and forming new memories.

Yes! You've guessed it! A compromised hippocampus can lead to difficulties remembering things like new names and faces.

It also makes it difficult to remember what you have already learned, like certain words, specific details, or the names of your old friends and classmates.

Well, you are not alone. Multiple studies have shown that this is a common frustration for many veterans who find gaps in their memories or struggle with learning new skills.

The Amygdala:

The *amygdala*, the part of your brain responsible for regulating emotions and activating responses to fear, may become overactive.

An overactive amygdala can make your world *seem* perpetually threatening, even when threats are minimal. This can turn even mundane interactions into sources of unexplainable anxiety.

When my boys were teens, they found great joy in sneaking up or hiding in the closet only to jump out and holler, "Boo!" To their delight, I all but leapt out of my skin.
I had an overactive amygdala. It's much better now. And my boys?

They no longer intentionally scare me, but it still happens, and when I startle for no apparent reason, they feel bad, but they still laugh. And I can live with that.

The Prefrontal Cortex:

Now, let's talk about your gorgeous *prefrontal cortex.*

The prefrontal cortex is involved in critical thinking and emotional regulation.

Like the hippocampus and amygdala, your prefrontal cortex may function less efficiently in response to constant stress.

When the prefrontal cortex is under constant stressors, you may experience a loss of emotional equilibrium.

You may suddenly feel overwhelmed, angry, or sad without understanding why.

In the context of PTSD and C-PTSD, the brain struggles to differentiate between past and present danger, keeping many of us locked in a state of hyperarousal or numbness.

This temporary state is more commonly known as the fight, flight, or freeze response. These responses are the brain's primitive way of protecting us from harm.

However, when the prefrontal cortex is over-stimulated, our responses may range from aggression and rage to panic attacks, crying, withdrawal, and dissociation.

Neuroplasticity

The concept of brain plasticity, or *neuroplasticity*, brings a shimmer of hope. This refers to the brain's ability to reorganize and form new neural connections throughout life.

This ability means that the injuries sustained from trauma are not necessarily permanent.

- ✓ **Simply stated: Recovery is possible!**

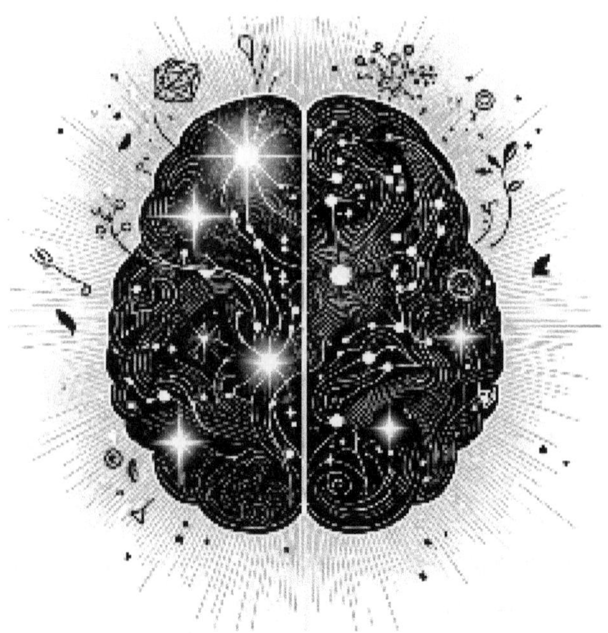

The brain can regain much of its lost function. For example, Therapies promoting relaxation and mindfulness stimulate the growth of the hippocampus, helping improve memory and reduce exaggerated stress responses by calming the amygdala.

Recovery strategies incorporating body-based therapies, mindfulness, and modalities that directly address the nervous system can be more effective than talk therapy alone.

For example, EMDR uses repetitive eye movements to help process and integrate traumatic memories and reduce their emotional impact over time.

For those wanting to take charge, kick-ass, and recover, neuroplasticity shines like a light at the end of a long and very dark tunnel.

This knowledge enables us to choose our treatment paths wisely. The concept encourages a holistic approach to actively engaging in approaches that support stress-impacted areas of the brain.

Holistic, self-help strategies can play a starring role in your recovery. Selecting activities that promote relaxation and mindfulness, such as yoga, meditation, or even simple breathing exercises, helps calm an overactive amygdala, making the world feel less threatening and more manageable.

Incorporating integrative approaches into your daily life isn't just about managing symptoms—it's about fundamentally understanding and mending the brain.

The research is clear. With patience and regular practice, we can indeed reclaim much of the control that trauma has taken from us. We will move forward. We will move from merely surviving to fully thriving.

The Body on Trauma

Trauma is not just a boogeyman of the mind. It also lingers in the body, manifesting through various physical symptoms that, at first glance, might seem unrelated.

When we speak of trauma, particularly C-PTSD, we often focus on the psychological scars. However, the body keeps its own score.

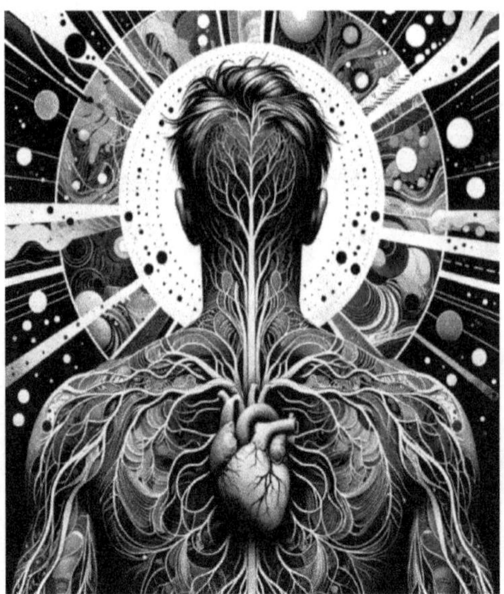

✓ **The body remembers moments of trauma, storing these memories in the muscles, the gut, and the heart rate.**

This is what we refer to as *embodied trauma*—a physical manifestation of psychological pain that strongly affects our health and well-being.

Consider how often we find ourselves dealing with unexplained physical ailments—aches and pains with no clear medical cause, gastrointestinal issues that arise during periods of stress, or the pervasive fatigue that no amount of sleep seems to cure.

Over 15 years ago, at the height of my military career, I was engaged in an extremely stressful leadership position. The operation tempo was high, and so were the stakes.

Out of the blue, I was hit with a sudden onset of migraine headaches. At first, it happened once a month, and then once a week, and then twice or thrice a week. It was nearly unbearable.

Then, less than a year later, a wave of debilitating and near-constant vertigo crashed down. Eventually diagnosed as *Meniere's disease*, vertigo stemmed from a dysfunction of the inner ear.

What caused these back-to-back, seemingly spontaneous maladies to wage war with a stressed-out but otherwise healthy young woman?

Without going into detail, I can count on two hands instances of abuse and trauma where I suffered minor to moderate brain injuries.

While neither the Migraines nor the Meniere's immediately followed such a traumatic event, both conditions are associated with traumatic brain injury. My little body had kept score. The logic leap here is over no great chasm.

Given this deep interconnection between body and trauma, integrating body-based therapies into your recovery process is not just beneficial. It is intuitively sound, allowing you to explore how trauma has settled into your body.

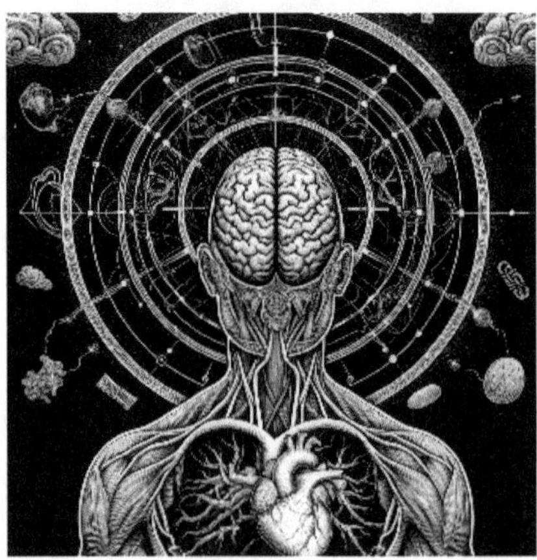

We must learn to tune into the body's signals. These little aches and pains are not our enemies. Instead, they are messengers guiding you towards areas that need care and attention.

The holistic approaches explored in the next chapters are about alleviating symptoms and fundamentally changing how your body responds to and holds trauma.

These strategies illuminate pathways out of the cycle of physical reactivity and into a state where recovery is not just a possibility. It's an ongoing activity.

Like any new practice, holistic approaches require patience and persistence. They involve relearning, recognizing, and tuning into the signals your body has been sending to communicate its distress.

As you become more fluent in your body language, you'll gain insight not only into your trauma but also into your intuitive ways of knowing how to speed your recovery.

Body-Based Approaches

Incorporating body-based therapies into your recovery process brings an acknowledgement that recovery is not solely a mental endeavor but a holistic one that involves the mind, body, and spirit.

This acknowledgement is key, for it aligns with the reality of how trauma operates, infiltrating every aspect of our being. By recognizing this, we can approach healing not as a segmented process but as a comprehensive nurturing of our entire selves.

Navigating the complexities of C-PTSD, where the wounds are deep and multifaceted, is about giving space for every part of you that has been affected—the mind, the body, and the spirit.

It's about building a dialogue between the three, fostering a relationship where each entity supports the healing of the other. This integrated approach improves symptoms and enhances overall quality of life, empowering you to move beyond survival to thriving.

As we explore these concepts, remember that the goal here is not to overwhelm but to offer insights and options. Each body is unique, and so is each pathway to healing. What works for one may not work for another, and that's perfectly okay.

The key is to listen—to *really listen*—to your body. Allow your body to guide you towards the theories and practices that somehow just *feel right.* This process is not about forcing a solution. Instead, it is about discovering tools your body resonates with, which will support your efforts to grow stronger and more resilient than ever before.

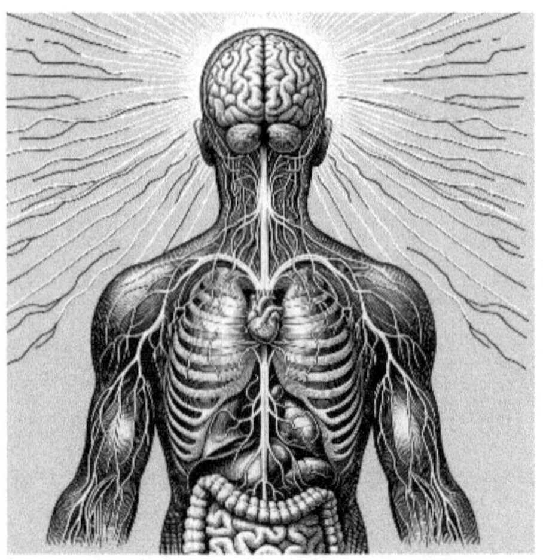

Polyvagal Theory: Understanding Your Nervous System

In the realm of understanding trauma's impact on our bodies and minds, the *Polyvagal Theory,* a model developed in 1994 by Stephen Porges, offers a revolutionary way to comprehend how our nervous system responds to stress and danger. More importantly, it provides a pathway to healing that is grounded in the biology of our bodies.

This theory has been particularly eye-opening for me and many others battling C-PTSD, as it shifts the narrative from one of enduring psychological distress to one of physiological adaptation and recovery.

At the heart of Polyvagal Theory is the *vagus nerve*, one of the longest nerves in the body. It plays a critical role regulating the heart, lungs, digestion, and even sexual arousal.

More than just a simple relay between the brain and body, the vagus nerve is pivotal in regulating our emotional landscape. It is interwoven in our experiences of stress and relaxation. It acts almost like pumping a car's brakes to slow down heart rate and calm internal systems.

This nerve is part of Porges' *parasympathetic nervous system*—the aspect of our *autonomic nervous system* that promotes rest and digestion, as opposed to the *sympathetic nervous system,* which prepares us to fight, freeze, or flee.

For those of us with complex PTSD, understanding the role of the vagus nerve is like finding a map in a dense forest. This map shows us how our bodies react to trauma, not just in immediate, short-lived moments but in long-term changes in how we process and respond to stress.

An underactive vagus nerve can mean our bodies are less able to return to a state of calm after stress, leaving us in a near-constant state of heightened alertness. This manifests in symptoms such as anxiety, sleep disturbances, and an inability to connect socially — all of which are common in C-PTSD.

Understanding our biology has significant power. Polyvagal Theory teaches us those feelings of safety and connection, called *social engagement*, stimulate the vagus nerve and shift our nervous system from defensive states.

This is where the concept of *safety* becomes not *just* a feeling. Safety becomes a physiological state.

When we feel safe, our bodies are more capable of readily activating parasympathetic responses, allowing for a reduction in heart rate, a calming of the breath, and a sense of peace that can be elusive for many who have experienced trauma.

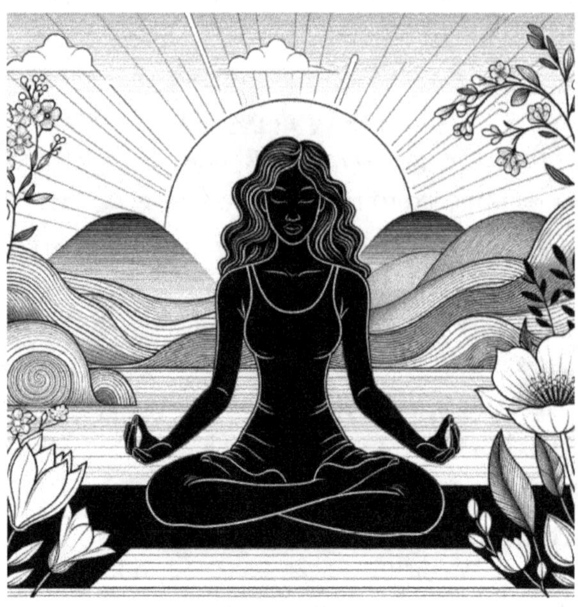

Applying the Principles of Polyvagal Theory in Everyday Life:

Creating spaces and relationships that foster feelings of safety and acceptance directly influence our nervous system, guiding it towards states of calm and healing.

This can be as simple as engaging in relaxing rhythmic activities like deep breathing, slow walking, or gentle yoga — practices encouraging the body to relax and the vagus nerve to release calming effects.

You can start applying these small, actionable steps:

1. Make time every morning for a few gentle stretches before starting your day.
2. Develop a practice of deep, slow breathing.
3. Choose gentle activities to move your body every day.
4. Regularly engage in social activities that feel safe and nurturing.

Incorporating the Polyvagal Theory into our recovery journey invites us to rethink our approach to healing from trauma.

It encourages us to consider the psychological and physiological pathways that can lead us toward recovery.

Polyvagal theory offers a holistic approach that respects and utilizes the innate wisdom of our bodies, fostering an environment where safety and connection pave the way for healing.

Complex PTSD in Women Veterans

While this next section focuses on military women with Complex PTSD, I urge you to keep reading. Knowledge is power. Besides, we can agree that both men and women, regardless of affiliation, may face some of the same dangers as military women.

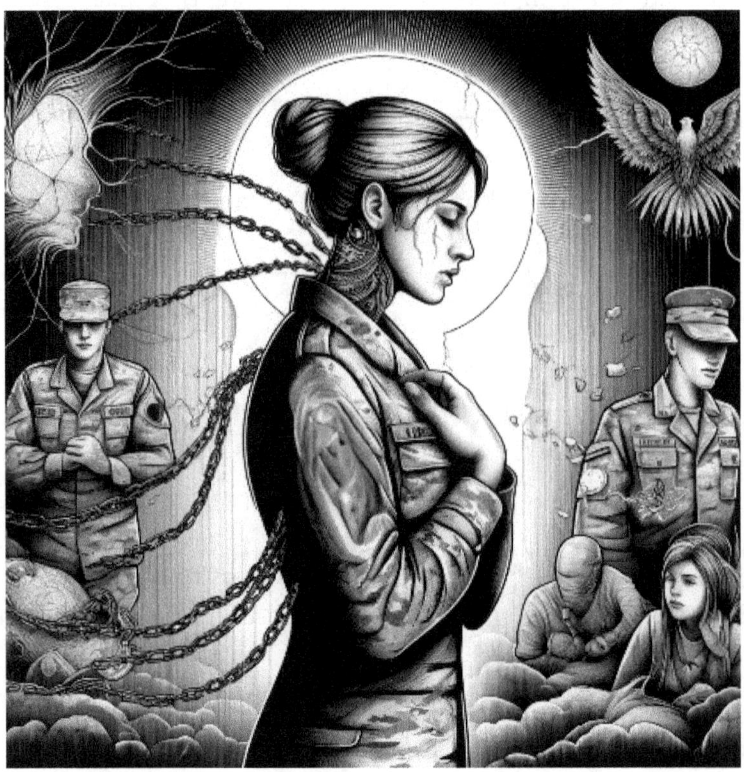

Abuses of power and *gender-specific trauma* can be found within the military ranks, on college campuses, and in our homes. You'll find it in boardrooms, factories, and workplaces worldwide.

The life of a woman serving in the military presents a unique set of challenges and experiences that can impact her mental health, particularly concerning complex PTSD.

Within the armed forces, women often face very specific traumas in hostile settings where they may feel powerless to remove themselves from the source of danger. These specific dangers include but are not limited to, military sexual trauma (MST) and pervasive gender-based discrimination—issues that can exacerbate the development of complex PTSD.

These experiences are not just about the events themselves. This is about how this brand of trauma alters a woman's perception of safety and trust and how these traumatic events are critically undermined in military environments.

Military sexual trauma, for instance, encompasses any sexual harassment or assault that occurs during military service. It's a harrowing reality that many women veterans have faced, often compounded by a culture that may discourage reporting such incidents due to fear of disbelief, retaliation, or damage to one's career.

The sense of betrayal is deepened when the perpetrator is a fellow service member, possibly someone whom the victim had to rely on for safety. This betrayal, coupled with the institutional hurdles that prevent many cases from being adequately addressed, can leave deep psychological scars.

Moreover, gender-based discrimination can manifest in many forms, from subtle biases in daily interactions to overt obstacles in career progression.

These experiences can contribute to a feeling of constant undervaluation and marginalization, reinforcing a sense of helplessness and isolation—fertile grounds for complex PTSD to take root.

The military, with its rigid hierarchies and emphasis on conformity, can often amplify these feelings, making it challenging for women to find supportive spaces within the system.

Recognizing the resilience and strength of women veterans is not just about acknowledging their hardships but appreciating their courage in navigating such a demanding environment.

Many women veterans carry their experiences with an admirable sense of strength and adaptability, qualities that are often overlooked. Their resilience is not just a testament to their individual characters but also a valuable asset in their recovery from complex PTSD. However, this resilience must be matched with tailored support and understanding, acknowledging the specific ways in which military experiences intersect with their psychological and physiological health.

The need for specialized resources and support networks for women veterans cannot be overstated.

Organizations like the Women Veterans Network (WoVeN) and the Service Women's Action Network (SWAN) provide essential support and advocacy for women who have served. These groups offer a range of resources, from legal assistance in cases of MST to mental health services tailored to the unique needs of women veterans. They provide spaces where women can share their experiences without fear of judgment, fostering a sense of community and mutual support that can be incredibly healing.

Wrapping it Up

Civilian and military mental health care are making great strides. The Department of Veterans Affairs (VA) is continually working on ways to address the needs of men and women diagnosed with PTSD.

The VA offers PTSD call centers for all veterans and recently included the *Women Veterans Call Center,* along with expanded services related to Military Sexual Trauma.

These resources are vital in helping our military veterans access the care and support they need, yet much remains to be done to address the scope of these collective yet very personal experiences.

The intersection of military service and complex PTSD in women veterans is a landscape marked by both challenges and remarkable resilience.

The military environment, with its unique stressors and structures, can deeply compound the effects of C-PTSD. However, recognizing the inherent strength of these women and men and providing them with tailored, empathetic support can pave the way for measurable healing and empowerment.

Moving Forward

As we continue pushing forward and building a greater understanding of the *brain-body connection* to trauma, we acknowledge our past.

We realize we are not defined by the past. We voice our rights to a life defined not by trauma but by our courage and resilience to face it.

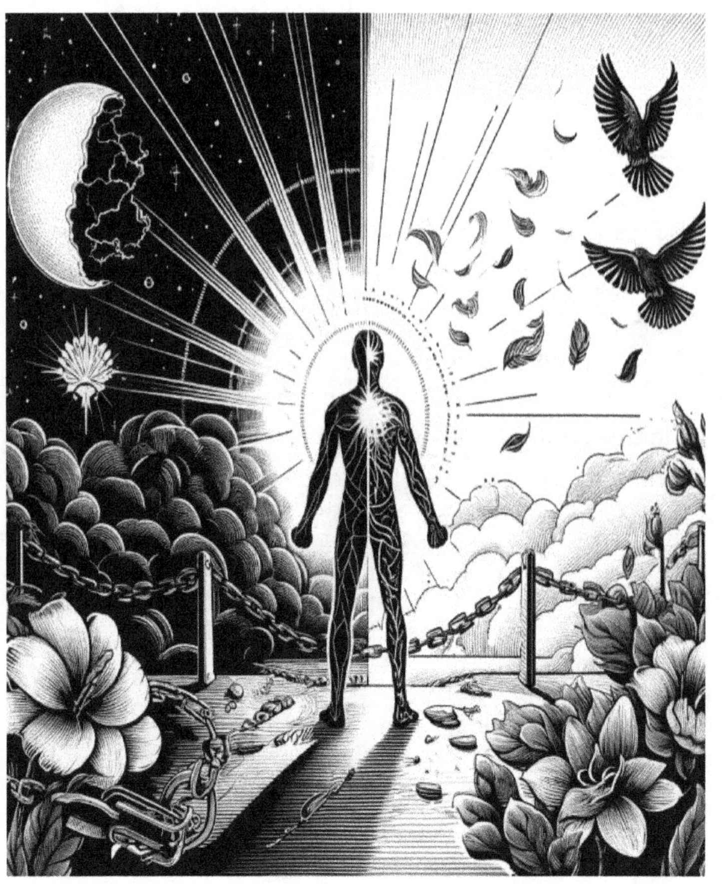

Step 3: Recognize Symptoms & Triggers

Imagine sitting in a coffee shop, enjoying a moment of peace. Suddenly, a door slams shut with a loud bang, and your heart starts racing uncontrollably. Your hands tremble, your breath quickens, and a flood of anxiety washes over you.

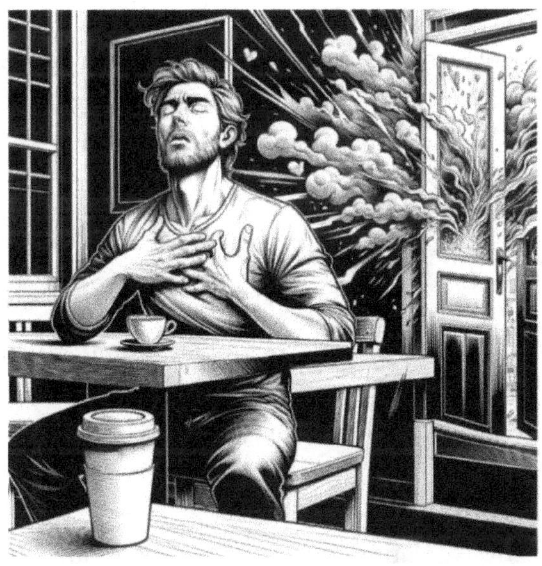

To an outsider, it may seem like a simple startle reflex, but for you, it feels like a full assault on your senses.

This is the complex world of PTSD symptoms—a world where it is not just the well-known flashbacks that haunt you but a spectrum of signs and responses that can transform ordinary moments into intense experiences.

Beyond Flashbacks: The Spectrum of PTSD Symptoms

When discussing PTSD, *flashbacks* often take center stage. However, the reality for many, especially those confronting C-PTSD, involves a far broader spectrum of symptoms that can permeate every aspect of life.

Learning to recognize and develop an understanding of your specific symptoms is a deeply important step. Your self-awareness and knowledge will help you craft a personal management strategy that encompasses the full range of your experiences.

Expanding the Definition:

Complex PTSD doesn't limit its influence on the overt re-living of past trauma. Instead, it extends its reach to how you regulate emotions, interact with others, and even how you view yourself.

Emotional dysregulation might manifest as sudden, intense bouts of rage, sadness, or irritation that seem, to the outsider, as overreactions to the situation at hand.

Avoidance behaviors are another common symptom, where you might find yourself steering clear of places, people, or activities that remotely remind you of past trauma. This drastically narrows your world.

An altered sense of self is particularly debilitating. You might feel disconnected from who you once were or struggle with a persistent sense of worthlessness. You may wonder if you'll ever feel 'normal' again.

Physical Symptoms

The physical manifestations of complex PTSD are often telltale signs of the disorder, yet these can be easily mistaken for other health issues.

Hypervigilance, for instance, might keep you constantly tuned in to your surroundings and on guard for potential dangers. As you are probably all too keenly aware, this makes relaxation seem like a foreign concept.

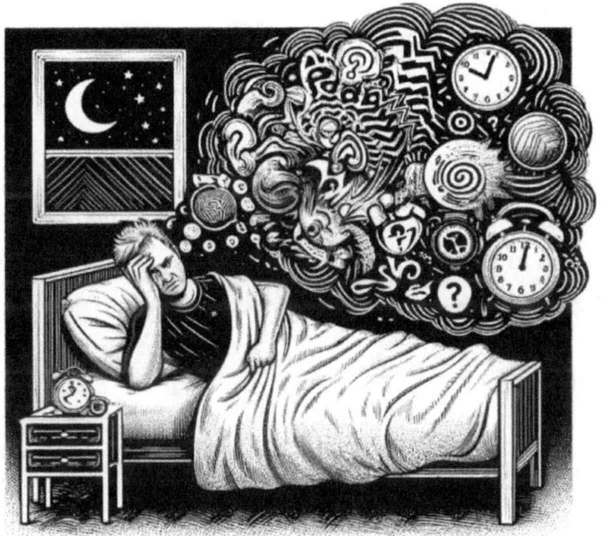

Insomnia can become a frustrating nightly battle, leaving you exhausted yet unable to sleep as your mind races with thoughts.

Somatic complaints such as unexplained aches, pains, and gastrointestinal problems are also frequent; these are not just random occurrences but are deeply tied to emotional distress, serving as physical reflections of inner turmoil.

Cognitive Effects

The cognitive effects of complex PTSD can be particularly challenging.

You might notice that your memory isn't as sharp as it used to be, with lapses that frustrate and scare you.

Difficulty concentrating can make everyday tasks feel overwhelming, impacting your productivity and self-esteem.

Intrusive thoughts might invade your mind, unbidden and unwanted, often at the least appropriate times, making it difficult to stay present in the moment.

These symptoms can create a vicious cycle where cognitive struggles reinforce feelings of inadequacy and anxiety, further exacerbating the condition.

Emotional Landscape

The emotional landscape of someone with complex PTSD can be fraught with intense, often conflicting emotions.

Shame and guilt, perhaps misplaced or irrational, can dominate your feelings and how you respond to these feelings.

These unchecked emotions are often compounded by a persistent sense of threat:

- The world doesn't feel safe anymore.
- You find yourself constantly on edge.
- You are waiting for the next bad thing to happen.

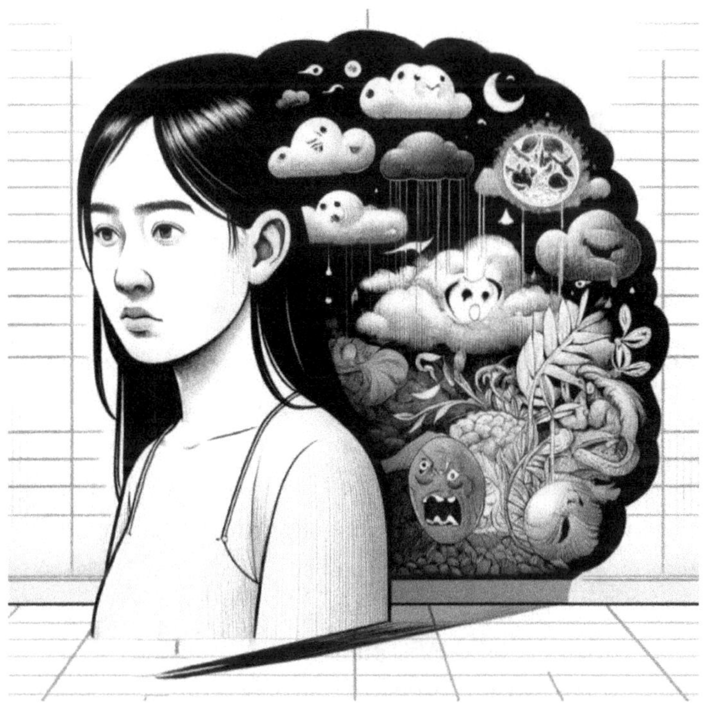

✓ **Operating in a state of chronic fear and sadness isn't just a series of emotional reactions but a condition that colors your entire perception of life.**

Textual Element: Reflection Section

To help you connect more deeply with the information shared and to foster a personal understanding of how these symptoms manifest in your life, consider reflecting on these questions:

- How do emotional dysregulation, avoidance behaviors, and an altered sense of self appear in my daily experiences?
- What physical symptoms have I noticed, and how might they be linked to my emotional state?
- Can I identify moments where cognitive effects have made daily tasks challenging?
- How do feelings of shame, guilt, and a persistent sense of threat influence my interactions and choices?

Reflecting on these questions can help you develop a more nuanced understanding of your symptoms, arming you with the knowledge to address them more effectively.

By acknowledging and exploring these various facets of complex PTSD, you can begin to reclaim control over your reactions and, ultimately, over your life.

This process isn't just about managing symptoms—it's about understanding them as integral parts of your story, which, when acknowledged, can lead to greater self-compassion and healing.

Identifying Your Personal Triggers

When navigating the complexities of C-PTSD, you must build an awareness of impulses that may trigger your symptoms. Triggers are specific stimuli—events, environments, people, or objects—that evoke intense emotional and physiological reactions to past trauma.

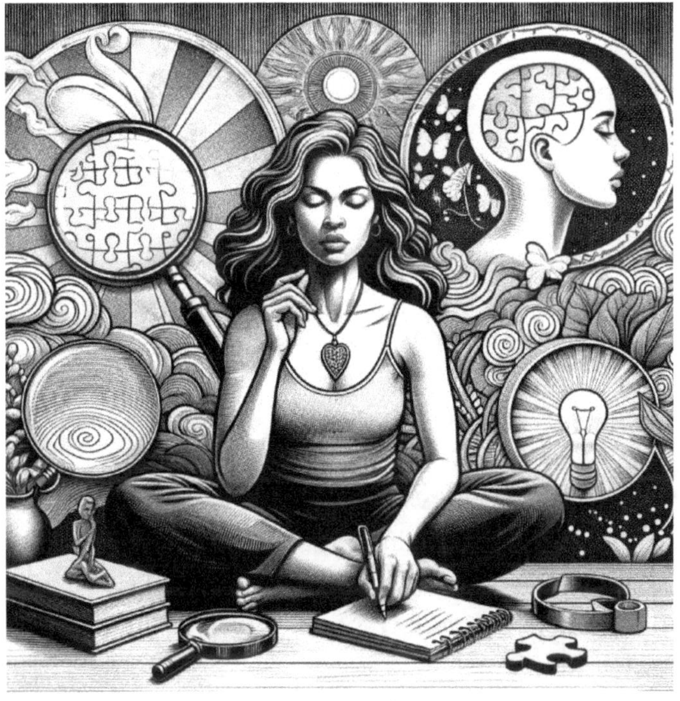

Triggers are deeply personal and can vary drastically from one person to another. For some people, a particular scent or sound will illicit memories of a traumatic event. For others, specific dates, locations, or even weather conditions cause discomfort or anxiety.

Identifying your personal triggers is much like detective work. It involves tuning in to your emotional and physical responses and tracing them back to their sources. This might sound straightforward, but it often requires deep self-reflection and mindfulness.

Journaling can be an invaluable tool in this process. By keeping a detailed record of when your symptoms escalate, you can begin to see patterns and identify potential triggers.

After experiencing a surge in anxiety, fear, or other intense emotions, take a moment of reflection to record the details.

Important! Please do not record details immediately following an episode. Wait until you know you are in a safe space.

Once you are ready, try asking yourself some of these questions:

1. Who were you with?
2. Where, exactly, were you?
3. What was happening around you when you first felt the surge?
4. Name the intense emotion. Was it fear? Rage? Sadness? Anxiety...?
5. List sensory stimuli, like sounds, smells, sights, taste, touch...
6. How close were you to the source of stimuli?

Learning to track anxiety, fear, or other intense emotions takes practice. You can create a voice journal using your phone or go old-school with pen and paper.

Please remember to approach this process with patience and compassion towards yourself. Creating a record can sometimes be challenging and triggering. This is why it is essential to wait until you are calmer and are in a place of safety.

Once you have a clearer idea of your triggers, you can map them out—a process known as *trigger mapping.* This involves creating a visual or written map outlining your identified triggers and the emotional and physical reactions these triggers provoke.

Your map can also include coping strategies you've found effective. The purpose of this map is not only to provide a visual representation of your triggers but also to help you predict and prepare for situations where you might encounter them again.

- ✓ **Trigger Mapping is a proactive approach, making disturbing situations more manageable and less daunting.**

Preventative Strategies to Lessen the Impact of Triggers:

Once you have identified and mapped your unique triggers, you can adopt coping strategies to lessen their impact.

One effective strategy is to develop *grounding techniques.* These techniques help you stay present, in the moment, and help you to disconnect from the emotional pain.

Examples of grounding techniques can range from deep breathing and mindfulness exercises to engaging your senses. Example: You can hold something cold, like an ice cube, or smell something familiar, like a favorite perfume.

One of my sensory grounding techniques is smelling a tangerine. I often keep one in my bag, especially whenever I fly. If ever I find myself in a busy marketplace, on the brink of feeling overwhelmed, I hit up the nearest fruit stand. Coffee beans work for me, too!

The key is to find grounding techniques that work specifically for you and practice them regularly so that they become second nature when you encounter a trigger.

Another essential strategy is creating a personal safety plan. This plan should outline actionable steps for you to take whenever you feel overwhelmed by triggers. These steps might include who to call for support, what environments feel safe, and which activities that help soothe you.

Having a plan in place provides a sense of control and safety, making it easier to navigate difficult moments. Communicate with your support network about your identified triggers and strategies for coping. Sharing this information can be daunting, but it can also strengthen your relationships and ensure that those around you know how best to support you in episodes of distress. Your network can also help hold space for you, providing a literal or metaphorical safe haven when triggers arise.

Understanding and managing your triggers is a dynamic process. As you change and grow in your recovery process, your triggers and how you respond to them will also evolve.

Regularly revisiting and updating your trigger map and safety plan can ensure that your coping strategies remain effective and relevant to your current state.

Trigger mapping is an ongoing commitment to self-awareness. Proactive management can substantially reduce the power that triggers may have over your life. Reducing trigger-power works while bolstering your own power to handle them will open up new spaces for healing and peace.

The Science of Memory and Trauma

When we consider the elaborate canvas of our memories, trauma acts like a thread that disrupts and distorts the pattern. Trauma weaves in confusion and fragments clarity once taken for granted.

Discovering trauma's impact on memory will help you understand why some of your memories seem disjointed or invasive.

Trauma significantly affects memory encoding and recall, leading to memories that are not neatly stored but fragmented and unpredictable in their re-emergence.

This results in memories that burst forth without warning, often triggered by seemingly unrelated events or sensations, capturing you in a moment of intense reliving.

These memories are not like the usual recollections of past events. Instead, they are visceral and loaded with all the original emotion and intensity, as if the past traumatic event is occurring in the present.

This phenomenon partly stems from how trauma can hijack the brain's normal memory processes.

Under typical conditions, the hippocampus helps form, organize, and store memories by placing them in a coherent context of time and space. However, under the duress of trauma, this process falters.

Stress hormones, particularly cortisol, overwhelm the hippocampus, impairing its function.

This disruption can prevent traumatic memories from being integrated into one's life narrative in the typical way.

Instead, these memories are often improperly processed and stored, making them feel current and exceptionally vivid whenever recalled.

Moreover, the intrusive nature of fragmented memories leads to considerable distress, as they often arrive without the usual narrative structure that helps differentiate past experiences from present reality.

This can make distinguishing between 'then' and 'now' particularly challenging. This may leave you feeling as though you're perpetually trapped in the moment of trauma.

False Memories and Distortions

Within the complexities of how trauma affects memory lies the potential for false memories or distortions. This aspect of memory science is fraught with controversy, especially concerning repressed memories—memories that are unconsciously blocked due to their distressing nature and later recalled.

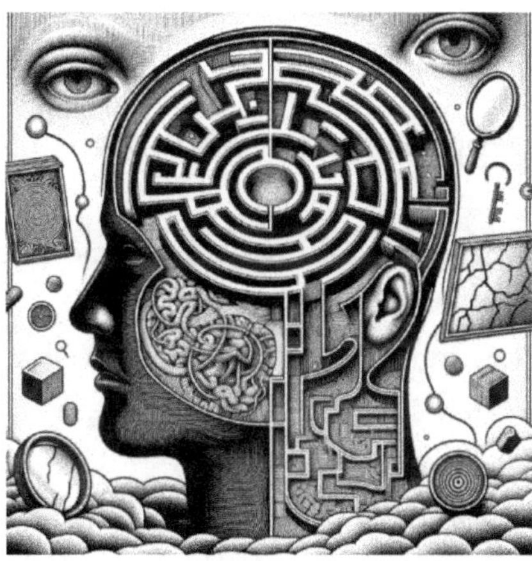

The debate surrounding false memories and distortions centers around the accuracy of these memories when they resurface, often during therapy or triggered by specific events.

This topic must be approached with care and sensitivity, as the implications can deeply affect someone's sense of reality and justice.

False memories arise from the brain's attempt to fill gaps in a fragmented memory narrative. This may occur when exposed to suggestive external influences, such as leading questions during therapeutic sessions.

These memories, whether partially or entirely inaccurate, feel incredibly real and emotionally charged.

Understanding the malleability of our memories, especially under the influence of trauma, is vital for those experiencing the memories and for professionals supporting a client's recovery. This highlights the need for therapeutic approaches that prioritize the careful handling of memory recall and emphasize the *emotional truth* of the experience over factual accuracy.

Therapeutic Approaches to Memory

Navigating the terrain of traumatic memories requires therapeutic approaches that respect the brain's altered state. These approaches must be applied gently to integrate these memories into one's coherent life narrative.

Narrative therapy, for instance, allows individuals to recount their traumatic experiences in a safe, structured environment, helping to restore context and perspective to fragmented memories.

Narrative therapy encourages you by repositioning *you* as the narrator of your own life story. The process provides a safe distance from the trauma and reduces its emotional impact.

As mentioned earlier, EMDR (Eye Movement Desensitization and Reprocessing) offers another powerful pathway in the realignment process.

This therapy involves recalling distressing images while receiving bilateral sensory input, such as side-to-side eye movements or hand tapping.

EMDR works by stimulating the brain's information processing system, helping transform the traumatic memory from a disruptive intrusion to an integrated, resolved memory.

This can substantially lessen the emotional pain associated with the memory, making it feel more like a narrative of a past event rather than a recurring event.

Memory as a Pathway to Healing

The journey through traumatic memories is not about erasing these experiences but about transforming how they live within you and how much space these traumatic memories take up in your daily life.

Integrating traumatic memories involves weaving them into the larger fabric of your life story, where they are acknowledged as part of your past but no longer have the power to dictate your emotional state.

This integration allows you to reclaim your life narrative and find meaning and strength in your survival and resilience.

It is worth noting that memory work requires courage and support because it involves revisiting painful and often terrifying moments. However, through therapeutic guidance and personal reflection, these memories can indeed shift from haunting presences to acknowledged chapters of your past, effectively reducing their impact and allowing space for new experiences and memories to form.

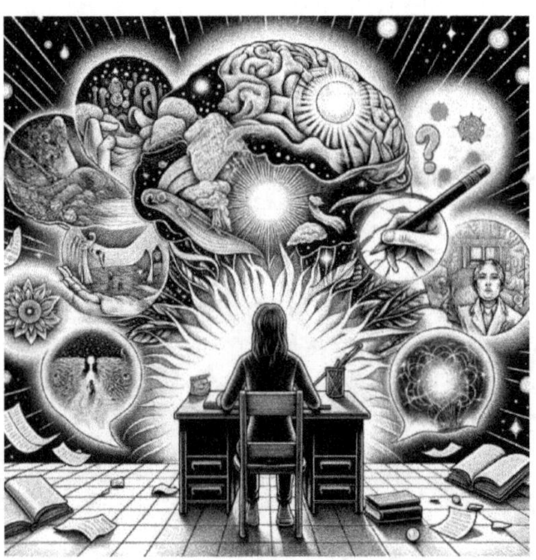

Memory work is an invaluable element in the C-PTSD recovery process, as it not only helps to alleviate symptoms but also contributes to a fuller, more capable sense of self.

By understanding and working through your memories, you will begin to control the narrative and, eventually, see your past with new clarity and embrace a future where trauma no longer holds the pen.

The Impact of Complex PTSD on Daily Life

Navigating the elaborate web of personal relationships may feel like a Herculean task when complex PTSD is part of your daily reality.

The extreme ways in which this disorder influences trust, intimacy, and communication may sometimes feel like invisible barriers, separating you from those you care about and those you wish to connect with.

Trust is the cornerstone of any meaningful relationship but often becomes compromised. You might find yourself constantly on guard. It's like having a silent alarm system that sets off by the slightest inconsistency or unfamiliarity, making it exceedingly difficult to let others in.

Intimacy, both emotional and physical, may also become fraught with anxiety. The vulnerability required to forge close connections can seem too great a risk, leading to a protective withdrawal into oneself. Others might misinterpret this withdrawal as coldness or disinterest.

Communication is also undoubtably affected. Expressing feelings and needs becomes tangled in a web of past experiences. Perhaps expressing your feelings once led to trauma. Or when you did express yourself, your feelings were dismissed, and your concerns were ignored.

You may find yourself constantly explaining and justifying your feelings.

Conversely, you might under-communicate by saying nothing at all in hopes of avoiding conflict or further misunderstanding.

These relationship challenges are not insurmountable, but they do require a conscious effort to navigate. It involves learning to slowly rebuild trust, not just in others but also in your own judgment of others. It's important to communicate openly about your experiences and boundaries.

C-PTSD and the Workplace:

In the professional realm, the impacts of complex PTSD manifest distinctly, influencing not just your productivity but your interactions with colleagues and your overall career trajectory.

Difficulty concentrating turns everyday tasks into overwhelming obstacles. Your mind might seem foggy as you struggle to focus on the task, leading to significant frustration and feelings of inadequacy.

Absenteeism may also become an issue, both physically and mentally—being present in a meeting while your mind replays a whirlwind of past traumas or worries.

Navigating workplace relationships can be challenging for anyone. However, the everyday stresses of professional interactions are amplified by complex PTSD. A simple critique from a supervisor might feel like a threat, triggering your fight, flight, or freeze response.

Moreover, complex PTSD deeply affects your self-perception and sense of identity. It may lead you to question your worth and abilities or view yourself through a distorted lens shaped by trauma. This altered self-perception often manifests as feelings of detachment or disconnection.

You might feel like you're going through the motions of your work, disconnected from the experiences and activities that used to bring joy or satisfaction.

This sense of detachment isn't limited to disassociating from painful memories or emotions. It may also extend to a general numbness, where your occupational highs and lows seem muted.

Lifestyle and Coping Mechanisms:

Adopted lifestyle and coping mechanisms by those living with complex PTSD vary widely and may be both adaptive and maladaptive.

On the adaptive side, you might find solace in routines and rituals that provide a sense of control and predictability.

Structured routines, whether morning exercises, scheduled social interactions, or designated times for relaxation and self-care, can provide an anchor, reducing feelings of chaos and unpredictability.

Maladaptive coping mechanisms may also emerge. These might include substance abuse, compulsive behaviors such as overeating, gambling, or self-isolation.

Initially, these newly adopted behaviors seem to offer temporary relief from emotional pain. Unfortunately, more often than not, these behaviors eventually exacerbate feelings of helplessness and isolation.

The daily life of someone grappling with complex PTSD stretches out in a landscape of varied and complex challenges.

Each aspect of life, from personal relationships to professional endeavors and self-concept, can be deeply colored by the symptoms of this condition.

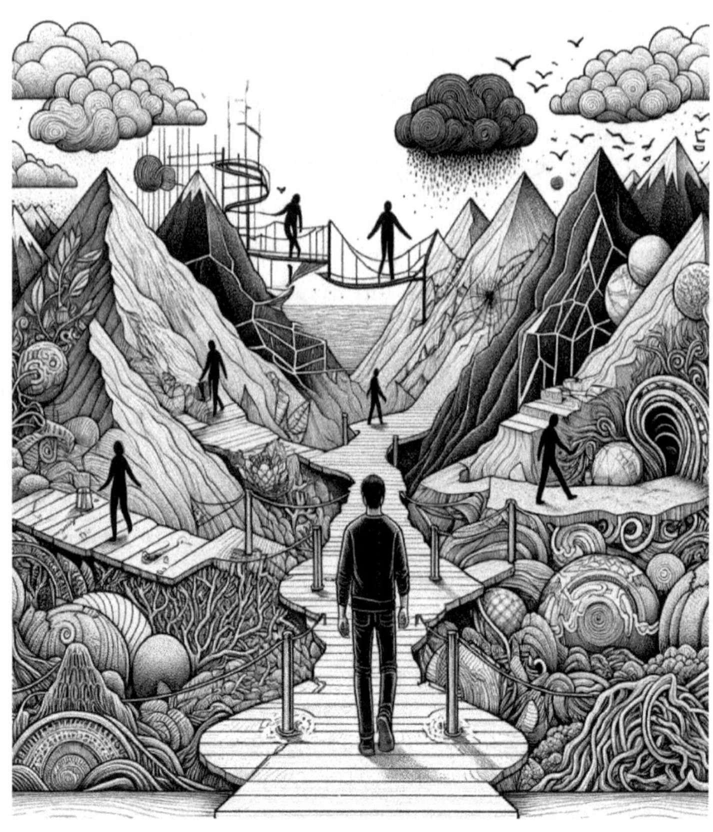

Dissociation: Strategies for Grounding

Dissociation in the context of complex PTSD is like an involuntary escape hatch your mind uses to protect itself from emotional overload. It's a psychological process where you might feel disconnected from your thoughts, feelings, or sense of identity.

In moments of dissociation, you may experience a sense of watching yourself from outside your body. Or you may find that the world around you seems unreal, like you're moving through a dream.

Dissociation is a coping mechanism that often develops in response to overwhelming trauma, serving as a form of mental retreat from pain.

Recognizing when you are dissociating might be challenging because the very nature of this response is to detach from your immediate reality.

Signs that you might be dissociating include the following:

- You are feeling numb or detached.
- You have a blurred sense of time.
- You experience the world in a distorted way.
- Sounds are muffled, and objects seem blurry.
- Key details of your day are hard to recall.
- You feel as if you are floating.
- You disconnect your emotions from the people around you.

Understanding these signs is the first step toward addressing dissociation, which will ultimately allow you to reclaim your sense of presence and reality.

Grounding techniques, like those mentioned earlier in trigger management, are also valuable when battling dissociation. These techniques bring you back to the here and now, reconnecting you with the physical world.

Mindfulness is especially effective in observing your current experiences without judgment. Mindfulness can be as simple as paying close attention to the sensations of your breathing or the sounds around you, anchoring you in the present moment.

Another powerful grounding technique involves deliberate and focused engagement of the senses. This method is often referred to as the *5-4-3-2-1 technique*. Here's how it works:

1. Identify five things you can see.
2. Locate four things you can touch.
3. Listen for three things you can hear.
4. identify two things you can smell.
5. Find one thing you can taste.

The 5-4-3-2-1 technique effectively redirects your attention from internal distress to external stimuli, helping to disrupt the dissociative state.

Integrating these simple grounding techniques into your daily routine will significantly enhance your ability to manage symptoms of dissociation.

Start by setting aside specific times each day for mindfulness practice, perhaps beginning with just a few minutes at a time.

Incorporating sensory engagement into your daily activities will also be helpful. For instance, you might choose a particular object—a smooth stone, a piece of soft fabric, a pack of gum, or even a tiny bottle of essential oil, like lavender—that you carry with you. Whenever you feel the onset of dissociation, focus on a texture, a taste, or a smell as your sensory anchor to ground you.

These strategies are not just about coping with dissociation; they are about enhancing your overall connection to the present and increasing your engagement with life.

By regularly practicing these techniques, you can reduce the frequency and intensity of dissociative episodes, making them less disruptive to your life. More importantly, you reclaim control over your internal state, enabling you to navigate your healing process with greater confidence and resilience.

Wrapping it Up

As we wrap up this chapter on recognizing symptoms and triggers, remember that understanding and managing these aspects of complex PTSD are foundational to your recovery.

In each section of this step, we have explored strategies, from trigger mapping to grounding practices. These strategies will help you manage dissociation and bolster your sense of personal agency and liberation.

Moving Forward

Our journey continues in the coming chapters as we shift our focus to holistic and integrative approaches that encompass the mind and the body. The next chapter will move deeper into Mindfulness, an approach that will further support your path to recovery, enhance your resilience, and increase your overall well-being.

Remember, each page you turn, each concept explored, and every step you take is an act of personal agency and an effort to reclaim your life from the shadows of trauma.

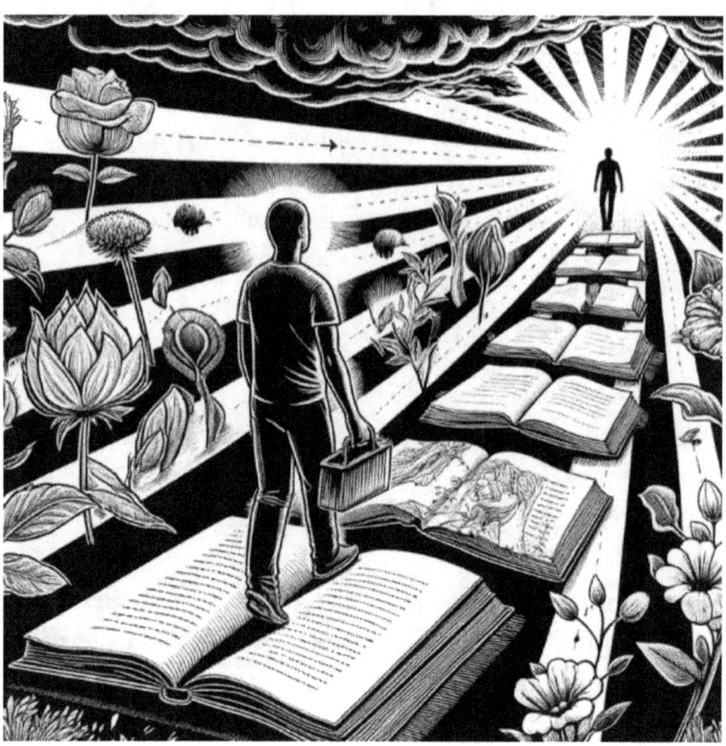

Step 4: Work Your Body

As we venture further into understanding the landscape of complex PTSD, particularly for those of us with military backgrounds, it becomes imperative to acknowledge the connection between our physical states and our emotional health.

This chapter explores somatic and physical therapies, which offer a powerful pathway to recovery as we focus on the body's role in trauma repair.

These approaches are not just about alleviating symptoms but are about engaging with the body in a way that promotes deep, lasting results.

The Power of Somatic Experiencing

Understanding Somatic Experiencing

Somatic Experiencing (SE) is a pioneering form of therapy developed by Dr. Peter Levine, aimed at resolving the symptoms of PTSD and other stress disorders through a focus on the body's physiological responses to trauma.

At its core, SE is about restoring the body's natural ability to regulate stress and restore equilibrium. It operates on the understanding that trauma disrupts our body's equilibrium, leading to a *freeze-response* that gets 'stuck' in our nervous systems.

The beauty of Somatic Experiencing lies in its gentle approach. Unlike some forms of therapy that require reliving traumatic events, SE works by helping you tune into your body's subtle cues and energies.

It's about noticing the sensations that arise when you recall a stressful experience and working through them in a slow, controlled manner. This process helps to release the pent-up *survival energy* that, when left unchecked, contributes to chronic stress, anxiety, and PTSD symptoms.

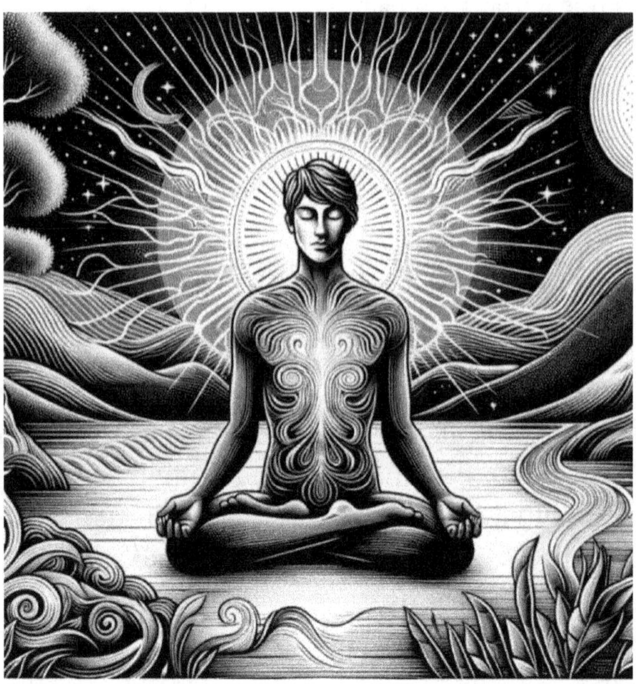

Principles of Somatic Experiencing

The foundational principle of SE is the tracking of bodily sensations. This involves observing the physical responses that occur in your body—tension, temperature, movement—and exploring these sensations without judgment.

The goal is not to change these sensations but to become aware of them, providing a way for the body to naturally recalibrate and recover.

Another core principle is *titration.* Titration refers to the process of slowly exposing yourself to the traumatic memory or trigger in small, manageable doses. By carefully and strategically not overwhelming the system, SE allows for the gradual release of stored trauma, making the process less distressing and more sustainable.

Self-guided Practices

While somatic experimenting is best conducted with a trained professional, there are aspects of it that may be safely explored on your own. Simple practices such as grounding and orienting are powerful tools.

Grounding involves practices that help you connect with the here and now, often through physical touch or attention to breath.

Orienting is the practice of slowly and deliberately noticing your environment with your senses, which helps you emerge from a traumatic flashback or dissociative state.

Try this simple exercise:

1. Find a comfortable place to sit or lie down.
2. Close your eyes.
3. Take a few deep breaths.
4. Focus on the sensations in your body.
5. Start with your feet.
6. Do you notice any areas of tension or discomfort?
7. Don't try to change positions to alleviate tensions or discomforts, just observe.
8. Now, slowly work your way all the way up to the very top of your head.

- ✓ **This practice helps increase body awareness, an essential first step in applying SE principles.**

Professional Support

While exploring SE on your own can be beneficial, working with a trained professional may provide deeper healing. A therapist trained in Somatic Experiencing guides you through the process and helps you navigate the more challenging aspects of trauma recovery. A professional offers support in managing intense emotions and sensations that arise, ensuring that the process remains safe and therapeutic.

Seeking a professional for Somatic Experiencing is a huge step in your healing journey. It's a commitment to addressing not just the symptoms of your trauma but its root causes. By working with a therapist, you will explore the depths of your trauma in a controlled and supportive environment, making it possible to find lasting relief and recovery.

Incorporating Somatic Experiencing into your recovery process invites a deepened engagement with your body's innate wisdom. It offers a path not just back to functionality but towards a deeper, more integrated sense of self.

As you learn to listen to and work with your body, you may find not only relief from symptoms but a new way of being in the world—a way that embraces the fullness of your experiences and the potential for renewal.

Therapeutic Yoga: Poses for Trauma Recovery

In the gentle embrace of therapeutic yoga, you find not just a series of poses but a nurturing pathway to reclaim your body's sense of calm and control after trauma.

The practice of yoga adapted for trauma recovery focuses on creating a safe internal environment where healing occurs. This safety is not merely about physical spaces but is more about fostering a sense of internal safety within your body—a fundamental aspect for those of us dealing with the aftermath of trauma, where feeling unsafe in our own bodies may be a persistent challenge.

Therapeutic yoga aids trauma recovery by encouraging a deep connection with the present moment through mindful movement and controlled breathing. This connection helps mitigate the disconnection from one's body that trauma often causes.

When you pay attention to your breathing and gently guide yourself through movements of intention and awareness, you also learn to recognize that your body is not the enemy.

With practice and patience, your body will become the most powerful ally in your recovery process. Your body is the tangible aspect of your being that you control and find joy in.

Your amazing body will separate itself from trauma, allowing you to take control of your physical sensations and reactions.

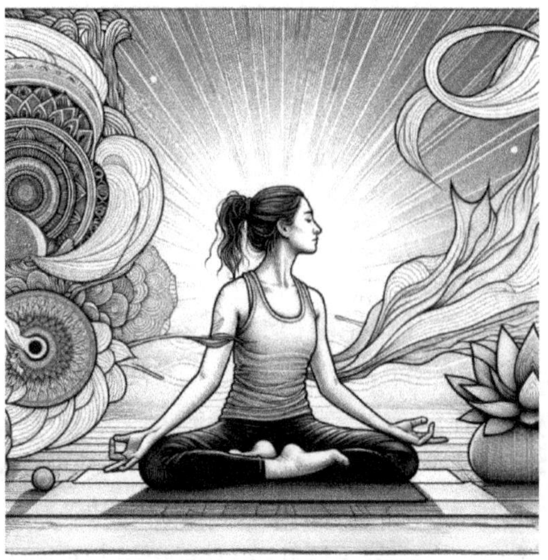

Therapeutic yoga includes specific poses and sequences that are particularly beneficial for releasing the physical and emotional tensions held in the body post-trauma.

Basic poses like *Child's Pose* offer a sense of grounding and safety, allowing you to curl up in a protective, nurturing way. This pose helps soothe the nervous system and is often used as a position of comfort during moments of overwhelm.

The Warrior series, on the other hand, is empowering, helping to build confidence and reclaim strength. These poses encourage a sense of resilience and personal power, qualities that are often diminished by traumatic experiences.

Another sequence that is highly beneficial involves gentle, restorative yoga poses combined with deep breathing. These poses are typically supported by props like cushions and blankets to ensure comfort and to help maintain the poses for longer periods. This practice allows for deep relaxation of the body, which leads to a release of long-held tensions and a significant reduction in symptoms related to anxiety and hyperarousal.

Creating a Safe Practice

When integrating yoga into your healing regimen, creating a safe and nurturing space is paramount. This space might be a quiet corner of your home where you feel comfortable and undisturbed.

Tips for Creating a Yoga Space:

- Make this space inviting and personal.
- Add soothing features like soft lighting, comforting scents, or calming music.
- Create a mini sanctuary with elements of nature: stones, crystals, or a small plant.
- Design a physical representation of the safe space you are trying to cultivate within yourself.

Modification and self-pacing are essential components of yoga practice, especially for trauma survivors. It's important to listen to your body and respect its limits.

Yoga is not about pushing yourself into poses but rather about finding a balance between comfort and gentle stretching. If a pose feels triggering or too intense, giving yourself permission to modify it or simply opt-out is not just okay—it's encouraged. Making choices based on your comfort level is a powerful exercise in rebuilding trust with your body.

Yoga instructors trained in trauma-sensitive yoga are particularly adept at guiding survivors through these practices with an emphasis on safety and choice.

A well-informed yoga practitioner will offer modifications for various poses and will often remind you that you are in control, that you can opt out of any movement that doesn't feel right, and that your well-being is the priority.

- ✓ **Please understand that sometimes, simply being present in the yoga space is a significant step toward your recovery.**

Engaging in therapeutic yoga is much more than physical practice. It's a holistic approach to healing that respects the deep connections between body, mind, and spirit.

As you continue to explore these practices, you may find that yoga provides not just relief from symptoms but also enhances your overall sense of well-being.

Your therapeutic yoga practice offers a path to gently reintegrate your physical self with your emotional self, bridging the gap that trauma often creates.

Through each pose, each breath, you're not just moving toward recovery; you're reclaiming your space in the world, one that is filled with calm, safety, and resilience.

EMDR:
Self-Administered & Professional

Exploring the realm of Eye Movement Desensitization and Reprocessing (EMDR) therapy, we uncover a tool to assist those of us grappling with the echoes of past traumas.

Originally developed by Dr. Francine Shapiro in the late 1980s, EMDR is a form of psychotherapy designed to alleviate the distress associated with traumatic memories.

Its effectiveness lies in its ability to help the brain process these memories, transforming them from haunting presences into integrated, manageable parts of one's narrative.

EMDR uses bilateral stimulation of the brain's right and left hemispheres.

This is typically done through guided eye movements, like the side-to-side movements of your eyes during the REM sleep phases. These guided movements assist with the natural processing of daily emotional experiences.

For many, the thought of revisiting traumatic memories is daunting. EMDR, however, approaches this gently.

By focusing on a traumatic memory while simultaneously experiencing bilateral stimulation, the vividness and emotion associated with the memory begin to fade. What remains is a memory that's less disabling, less vivid, and far less disturbing.

Think of EMDR therapy as removing the sharp spines from a cactus. Once you remove the prickly parts, the shape and color remain. However, those prickly parts can no longer hurt you as much as they once did.

While EMDR is typically performed under the guidance of a trained therapist, there are principles from this therapy that may be adapted for personal use, particularly for managing stress and minor triggers.

These self-administered techniques should not replace professional therapy but serve as additional tools in your coping arsenal.

One such technique is to give yourself a *Butterfly Hug.* Feel free to give yourself a hug right now.

Follow these easy steps:

1. Cross your arms over your chest.
2. Rest your hands on your upper arms.
3. Alternately tap your upper arms with the tip of your fingers.

Did you try it? Oh, good. Wasn't that nice?

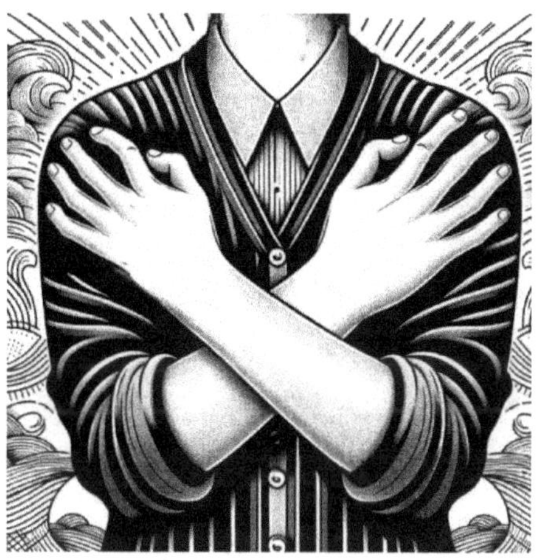

The Butterfly Hug is just one very simple DIY hack to mimic the bilateral stimulation used in EMDR. It might be soothing whenever you are feeling overwhelmed.

I started using the Butterfly Hug several years ago while teaching in Japan. I needed a portable, easy-to-employ coping strategy while riding public transportation.

The trains in Tokyo are crowded and often overwhelming, but I'd find a seat or something to lean against and give myself a little therapeutic hug.

Another DIY technique is walking with trekking poles. I discovered this quite by accident while on pilgrimage. The slow, rhythmic movements and the tap-tap-tapping of the poles works to connect the right and left hemispheres of the brain and can be very soothing.

Limitations and Precautions

While these techniques offer temporary relief and a greater sense of control over your emotional state, they have their limitations. Self-administered EMDR techniques are not a substitute for professional EMDR therapy, especially for those with complex PTSD and severe trauma histories.

The depth and intensity of such traumas often require the safety and structure of a therapeutic relationship, where a trained professional guides the process and handles any intense reactions that might arise.

Please approach self-administered techniques with a healthy blend of curiosity, optimism, and caution. If at any point you find your emotional reactions are intensifying or you feel an overwhelming resurgence of traumatic memories, take this as a signal to cease these practices and seek professional guidance. The goal of using these techniques is to manage stress and minor triggers, not to unpack deep-seated traumas alone.

Resources for Finding EMDR Therapists

If you want to explore professional EMDR therapy, several resources will help you find qualified therapists. *The EMDR International Association (EMDRIA)* website offers a therapist locator to find certified EMDR therapists based on location. Additionally, many mental health professionals now include EMDR as part of their therapeutic offerings, and their profiles often mention their certification levels.

Another valuable resource is the *Psychology Today* therapist directory, which allows you to filter therapists by those specializing in EMDR. Here, you may also read about each therapist's approach and other areas of expertise, ensuring you find someone whose style and qualifications meet your needs.

- ✓ **Seeking support through EMDR therapy can be a major step toward healing. It's an acknowledgment that while the journey has been tough, the strength and resilience within you are tougher.**

As you consider these resources and perhaps begin to reach out, remember that seeking help is a sign of courage. Each step, whether self-administered practices or reaching out to a therapist, is a move toward a more grounded and peaceful you.

The Benefits of Regular Exercise on PTSD

Embracing the rhythm of your breath as you move and feeling the pulse of your heartbeat aligns you not just with your body but also with a sense of being alive, present, and engaged. This is the essence of using regular exercise as a recovery tool for PTSD.

Studies have consistently shown that engaging in physical activity significantly alleviates symptoms of PTSD by reducing anxiety levels, decreasing the occurrence of depressive episodes, and enhancing overall mood stability.

The release of endorphins, often called the body's natural painkillers, during exercise plays a critical role in this process. These powerful biochemicals promote an immediate sense of well-being and, over time, contribute to a sustained improvement in overall mental health.

For those of us navigating the complexities of PTSD, the types of exercise we choose will be as varied as our experiences. Cardiovascular exercises such as running, cycling, swimming, rowing, or even brisk walking have a dual benefit. They not only improve physical health but also help reduce hyperarousal symptoms.

The rhythmic, repetitive nature of many cardio exercises, like the elliptical machine at the gym or hiking with trekking poles, is a form of moving meditation. These rhythmic movements provide a mental break from intrusive thoughts, allowing us to focus on the bodily sensations that anchor us in the here and now.

Strength training, on the other hand, may empower you by reinstating a sense of control over your body. Lifting weights or engaging in resistance training exercises helps build not just muscle but also confidence and personal agency, qualities that trauma often diminishes.

Group sports or classes, like soccer, softball, water aerobics, or dance, are particularly therapeutic. These settings offer not just physical benefits but also a chance to connect with others. This fosters a sense of community and belonging. When faced with the isolation tendencies of PTSD, these social interactions provide a support network that shares the unspoken bond of striving towards better health, both mental and physical.

Participating in group activities and team sports also enhances motivation and commitment to regular exercise, making the whole experience more enjoyable and sustainable.

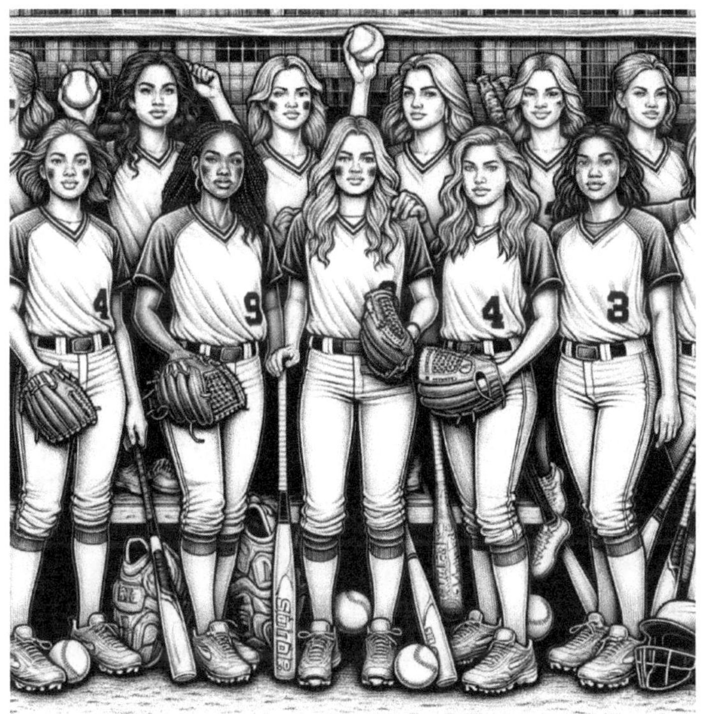

Setting realistic goals is fundamental in making exercise a part of your healing process. Recognize where you are, both physically and emotionally. Starting with overly ambitious goals may lead to frustration and setbacks, which might deter further participation. Instead, set achievable, incremental goals. This will foster a sense of accomplishment and encourage persistence.

If you are new to exercise or returning after a long sabbatical, you might start with a goal of walking for 10 minutes a day. Gradually increase your walking time as you feel more comfortable and confident.

Remember: ***Your best is good enough*****!**

Some days might be harder than others, and that's perfectly okay. What matters is showing up for yourself, in whatever capacity you are able.

Integrating exercise into your daily life need not be a daunting task. One effective strategy is to incorporate physical activity into your existing routines. For example, if you spend a significant amount of time commuting, consider biking or walking part of the way.

Simple changes, like taking the stairs instead of the elevator, increase your daily activity levels without requiring too much additional time or effort.

Another helpful approach is to plan your workouts ahead of time. Just as you might schedule a meeting or a doctor's appointment, scheduling your exercise sessions will help ensure that movement becomes a non-negotiable part of your day.

For those times when motivation wanes, as it naturally might, having a backup plan will make a big difference. This could be as simple as rolling out a yoga mat in your living room for a quick session or having a set of dumbbells within easy reach for lightweight lifting. The key is to make it as easy as possible to choose an active option, especially on days when your energy or motivation might be lower than usual.

Engaging regularly in physical activities offers a pathway to improved physical health and emotional and psychological recovery.

The discipline and focus required to maintain a regular exercise regimen provides a constructive outlet for the frustrations and challenges that come with PTSD. More importantly, it reminds you of your strength, resilience, and ability to persevere—qualities that define you much more than your trauma.

As you continue to integrate exercise into your life, let each step, each lift, and each cha-cha-cha celebrate your commitment to not just surviving but also thriving.

Integrating Breathwork into Your Healing Journey

Let's turn our focus towards an often overlooked yet potent tool in managing PTSD: *Breathwork*. This simple yet significant practice centers on controlling your breath to influence your mental, emotional, and physical states, providing a direct pathway to soothe your nervous system.

For those of us confronting trauma, learning to harness the power of our breath offers a readily accessible resource for self-regulation and calm anytime and anywhere.

Breathwork operates on a basic principle: ***By changing the patterns of your breathing, you alter your emotional and physiological state.***

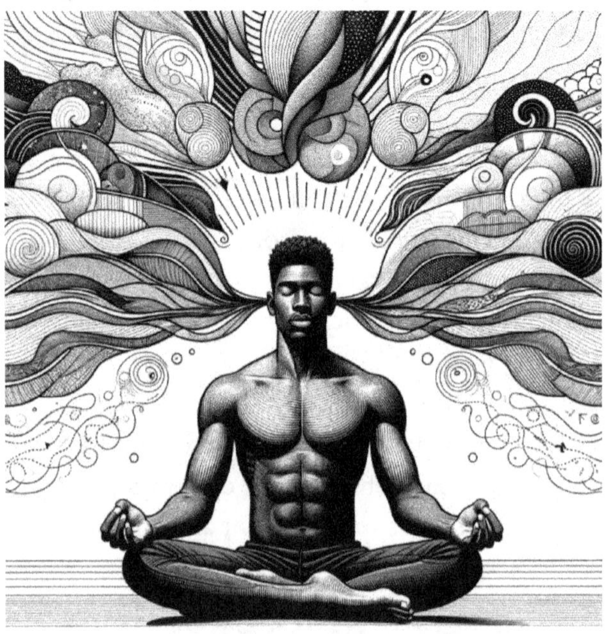

When you experience stress or recall a traumatic memory, your breathing becomes quick and shallow.

This is a part of the body's natural fight-or-flight response. This type of breathing will amplify feelings of anxiety and disconnection.

However, deliberate, deep, and rhythmic breathing shifts your body's balance towards relaxation and grounding, reducing the immediacy of stress and creating a sense of presence that anchors you firmly in the here and now.

Engaging in deep breathing exercises stimulates the *vagus nerve.* As we learned in Step 2, the vagus nerve is a critical component of the parasympathetic nervous system, which oversees an array of important bodily functions, including mood regulation and stress levels.

Activating your vagus nerve through deep breathing techniques decreases heart rate and blood pressure, fostering a state of calm throughout the body. Furthermore, controlled breathing increases the supply of oxygen to your brain and stimulates the production of endorphins, the body's natural painkillers. This enhances both your mood and overall sense of well-being.

If you are new to this practice, several simple techniques are easily incorporated into your daily routine.

You might like to give the 4-7-8 Breathing Method a try:

1. Inhale through your nose for four seconds.
2. Hold your breath for seven seconds.
3. Slowly exhale through your mouth for eight seconds.

The 4-7-8 technique acts as a natural tranquilizer for your nervous system, providing a quick and potent means of reducing anxiety and regaining emotional equilibrium.

Another helpful practice is *Diaphragmatic Breathing,* which involves deep breathing that engages the diaphragm, allowing the lungs to expand fully. This fosters a deep sense of relaxation.

Go Ahead! Give Diaphragmatic Breathing a Try:

1. Lie on your back.
2. Put one hand on your belly and the other on your chest.
3. Breathe deeply.
4. Focus on making your belly rise more than your chest.
5. Continue your process until you notice a significant relaxation response.

Incorporating breathwork into your life need not be a cumbersome addition to your schedule. It may be seamlessly integrated into your existing routines. For instance, taking a few minutes each morning to practice deep breathing will set a calm tone for the day ahead.

Using breathwork techniques during transitions between daily activities—such as shifting from work tasks to personal time—can help manage stress and maintain a steady emotional state throughout the day.

Consider using breathwork as a reactive tool; when you feel symptoms of PTSD arising, such as heightened anxiety or flashbacks. Take a moment to engage in deep, controlled breathing. This helps mitigate these symptoms, returning you to a calmer and more functional state.

Breathwork not only offers immediate relief but also contributes to your long-term recovery goals. Regular practice helps train your body and mind to default to deeper, more calming breathing patterns. This gradually diminishes the intensity and frequency of PTSD symptoms.

Breathwork encourages a deeper connection with your body, enhancing your ability to listen to and respond to its needs with care and understanding.

This exploration of breathwork as a healing tool emphasizes the theme of holistic recovery that we've been exploring throughout this chapter.

Whether through the grounding practices of Somatic Experiencing, the liberating poses of therapeutic yoga, the transformative process of EMDR, or the vigorous release of regular exercise, each modality offers unique benefits that contribute to a comprehensive approach to healing.

Breathwork ties all these practices together, providing a simple yet powerful technique for enhancing bodily awareness and emotional regulation, which are essential components of the recovery process.

Wrapping it Up

As we close this chapter, remember that the journey to recovery is not linear. Instead, it is a path marked by exploration, learning, and growth. Each step forward, no matter how small, is a victory in reclaiming your life.

As you continue to integrate these various therapeutic practices, you will find not just relief from symptoms, but a deeper and more joyful engagement with life itself.

Moving Forward

In the next chapter we will dive deeper into creative and expressive therapies. We'll explore how activities like art, music, pottery, and writing serve as vital outlets for self-expression and processing traumatic experiences.

These therapies offer not just healing but also a way to reclaim and rediscover parts of yourself that may have been overshadowed by trauma.

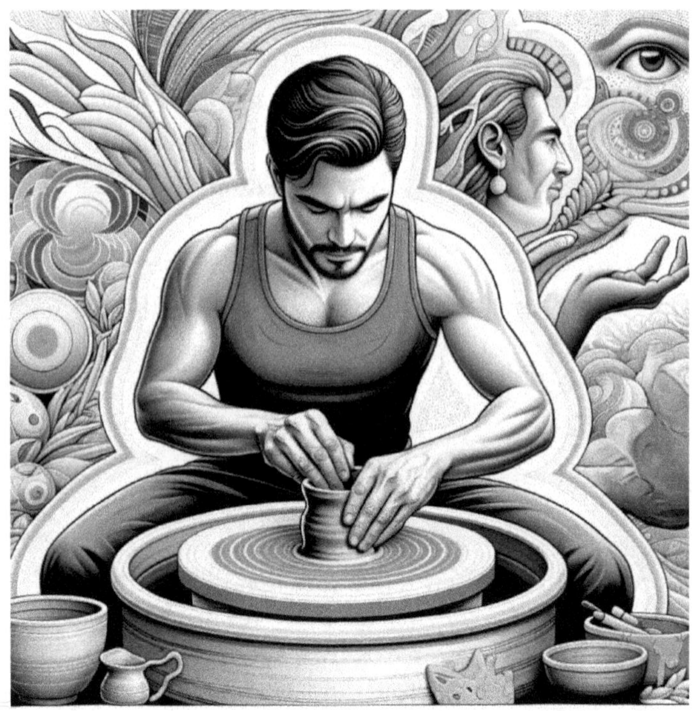

Join me as we explore these creative pathways to recovery, each offering new opportunities to weave resilience and joy back into the fabric of your life.

Step 5: Be Creative!

In the complicated mosaic of recovery, each tiny piece plays a pivotal role in crafting the overarching picture of wellness. Creative and expressive therapies represent vibrant and essential pieces of this mosaic, offering you a unique pathway to express and process feelings that words alone cannot.

As we dig into these therapies, imagine each stroke of the brush, each line on a page, as a step towards not just understanding your trauma but also transforming it into something more, something uniquely yours. Here, in the realm of colors, shapes, and textures, your experiences are validated, and your emotions find a safe harbor for expression.

Art Therapy:
Drawing Your Path to Recovery

Art therapy emerges as a beacon for many who find traditional verbal expression challenging. It provides a canvas where emotions and memories are externalized, examined, and understood through the varying mediums of art.

This form of therapy harnesses the power of creativity to facilitate healing and personal growth, allowing you to communicate what may be too difficult to express with words. The process of making art will help you to externalize and organize your thoughts, which is particularly therapeutic for those struggling with the scattered memories and intense emotions characteristic of C-PTSD.

One of the benefits of art therapy lies in its ability to access and process traumatic memories in a non-verbal way. Trauma often leaves you feeling wordless. Sometimes, the experiences are too overwhelming for speech.

Art acts as a mediator, allowing you to express these feelings safely and tangibly. This expression may be immensely relieving, especially when emotions feel congested inside. As you paint, draw, sculpt, or work behind the potter's wheel, you are essentially unpacking the burden of these emotions, placing them outside yourself where they will be seen and transformed.

If you are looking to explore art therapy on your own, several simple activities may be undertaken at home. You might begin with something as straightforward as a *color feelings chart*, where different colors represent different emotions.

Try a Color Feelings Chart:

1. Select colors that resonate with how you feel in the moment.
2. Use these colors to fill up the page.
3. While filling up the page, reflect on your choices.
4. Yes! It is that simple.

- ✓ **The act of choosing and applying color is a revealing reflective process.**

Another simple activity involves creating a trauma narrative through collage:

- Find images from magazines or newspapers that resonate with your experiences.
- Arrange these images to tell your story.

Creating a narrative collage helps externalize and organize your thoughts. This is just one way to help you communicate about your past experiences.

Finding a qualified art therapist will significantly enhance your journey through art therapy. When searching for a therapist, look for credentials such as registration with the *American Art Therapy Association*, which ensures they have the necessary training and experience.

During art therapy sessions, expect a supportive environment where you are encouraged to explore and express your emotions through various art forms. The therapist will guide you through the process, helping you to interpret your artwork and understand your emotional responses, facilitating deeper insights into your experiences and feelings.

Art therapy also serves as a powerful tool for self-discovery and personal development. It's not merely about creating something pleasing to the eye; it's about letting your inner world manifest in visual form.

Through this creative process, you might discover new aspects of yourself, uncover hidden emotions, or come to terms with aspects of your past.

This fosters greater self-awareness and acceptance. These are valuable steps toward recovery.

As you engage with art therapy, allow yourself to be open and honest in your creative expression. There is no right or wrong way to create art in this context. It's all about what feels true and healing for you.

Let each choice of color, each mark on the paper, be a step towards reclaiming your narrative and healing your spirit. In this space, you are free to explore, free to express, and free to heal, all guided by the gentle power of your own creativity.

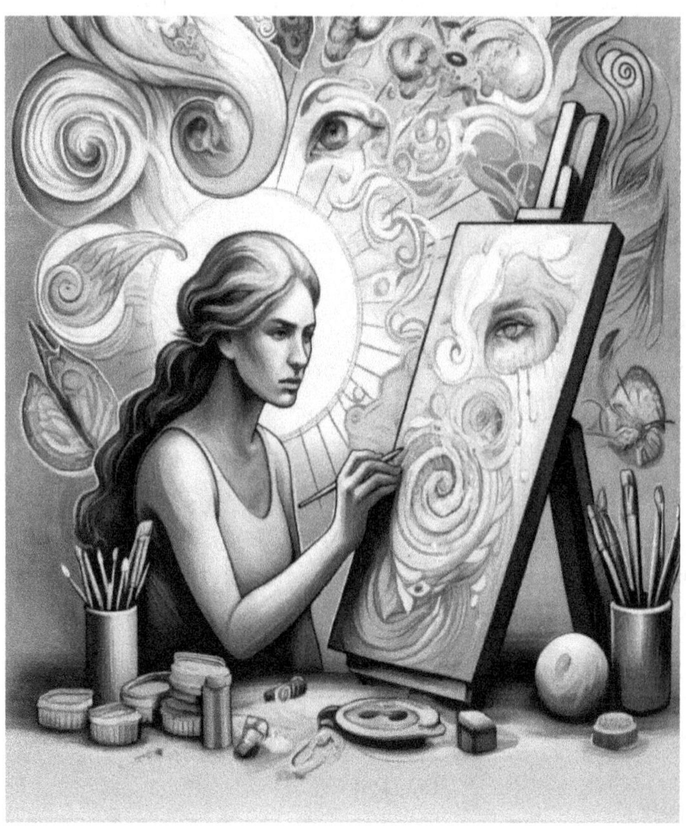

Writing for Healing: Journaling and Beyond

Grasping a pen, feeling its weight, and seeing your thoughts spill out onto paper is often a pivotal moment in healing. This process, known as therapeutic writing, extends beyond mere documentation. It involves a deep, reflective dialogue with oneself, providing a unique avenue to articulate and process complex emotions and memories tied to trauma.

- ✓ **The act of writing helps externalize those thoughts and feelings that may feel too overwhelming or difficult to speak about.**

Finding a way to get those words out is like setting down a heavy load you've been carrying. Once the words are out in the open, you might examine them from different angles and eventually find a way to let them go or learn to carry them more comfortably.

Therapeutic writing encompasses a variety of forms, each offering distinct benefits. Journaling is perhaps the most straightforward of these. Journaling involves regular, often daily, entries that capture your thoughts, feelings, and experiences. This practice serves as a powerful tool for emotional catharsis and self-reflection.

Writing down what you are going through helps organize chaotic thoughts and provides clarity. Sometimes, seeing your feelings in writing makes them more manageable and less intimidating.

This can be incredibly soothing. Moreover, journaling creates a chronological record of your thoughts and feelings, which may be extremely helpful in tracking patterns or triggers over time, aiding in both self-understanding and therapeutic interventions.

To guide you in this practice, consider these journaling prompts designed to help you explore your thoughts, feelings, and trauma narratives safely and compassionately:

1. **Today I felt...** - Begin by simply acknowledging your feelings without judgment. Whether it's sadness, anger, joy, or a mix of many emotions, write them down.
2. **A situation that challenged me today was...** - Reflect on difficult moments and explore why they were challenging.
3. **One thing I did well today...** - Recognize and celebrate your daily victories, no matter how small they may seem.
4. **I felt most like myself when...** - Identify moments or activities during the day when you felt most in tune with yourself.

Expanding beyond journaling, creative writing offers another therapeutic outlet. This form of writing allows you to use poetry, stories, or letters to express and process emotions.

Poetry is particularly effective as its metaphorical language allows for the expression of nuanced feelings and experiences that might be hard to articulate in prose.

Writing stories, on the other hand, offers a means of exploring different perspectives, perhaps imagining a situation from another's viewpoint, which fosters empathy and a deeper understanding of one's own reactions.

Letters written to yourself or others (regardless of whether you send them or not) are ways to articulate feelings, experiences, and forgiveness in a direct, personal format.

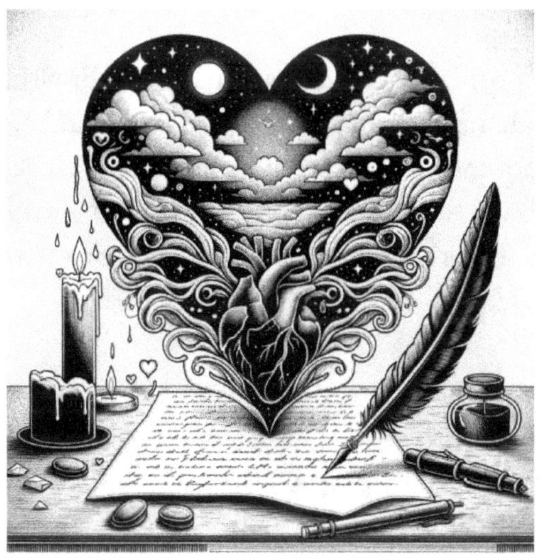

These creative avenues often reveal insights and understandings that might remain elusive in more direct analyses of your experiences.

Before engaging in therapeutic writing, please consider your privacy concerns and personal boundaries. The intimate nature of this work means it may sometimes bring up deeply personal and potentially distressing memories and emotions.

It is important to create a safe space for your writing practice. This might mean keeping your journal in a private, secure place or setting clear boundaries with yourself about what topics you are ready to explore.

Remember: You are in total control of the pace and the depth of your expression and exploration. If a particular topic or memory becomes too overwhelming, it is perfectly okay to step back and either leave it for another time or choose not to write about it at all.

If you are considering sharing any part of your writing, whether with a therapist, a friend, or a wider audience, think carefully about what feels safe to share and what you prefer to keep private. Sharing is a powerful act of vulnerability and trust, but it should never come at the expense of your emotional safety.

Therapeutic writing, in all its forms, offers a way to navigate the complexities of healing from trauma. It provides a private, controlled environment where you confront and make sense of your experiences at your own pace.

Whether through the structured lines of a journal, the flowing verses of a poem, or the narrative of a personal story, writing allows you to reclaim your voice and tell your story. The act is transformative because you can rewrite the outcome of trauma. You can change trauma from an episodic telling of what happened into a narrative of survival and resilience.

- ✓ **Yes! You have the power to choose your words and write yourself a better ending.**

As you continue to write, remember that each word you pen is a step towards understanding, healing, and reclaiming the narrative of your life.

Music as Medicine: Playlists for Emotions

Music holds an almost ethereal quality, with the power to shift your mood, evoke deep memories, and even alter your perception of time and space. It's like a universal language that speaks directly to the soul, bypassing the need for words, making it a valuable tool for emotional regulation and healing.

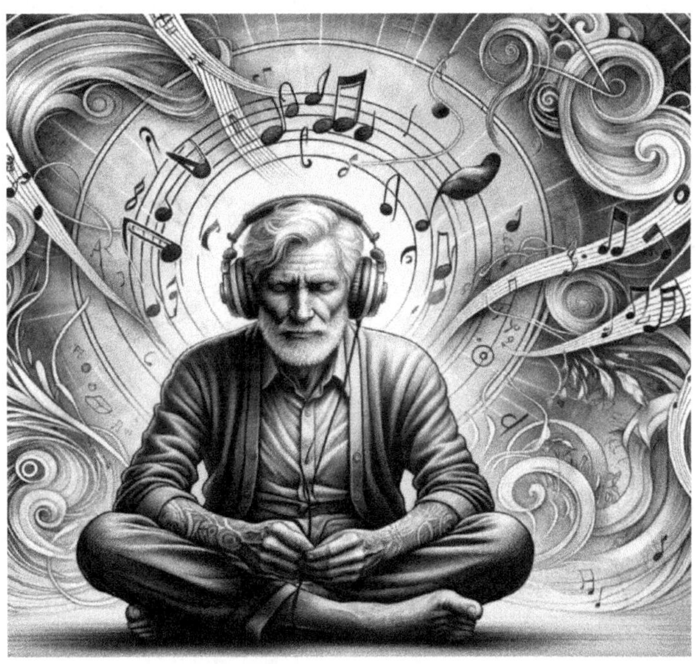

Music might be your therapeutic ally, helping you to manage the intense emotions and mood fluctuations that often accompany C-PTSD. Using music intentionally to regulate mood involves understanding how different types of music affect your emotional state and using this knowledge to create a sound environment that supports your emotional needs.

Imagine you're in a busy restaurant. It's too loud, and you're feeling anxious. Your thoughts are racing, and your heart is pounding. And then, suddenly, from the speaker above you, you hear a familiar song. You recognize the melody instantly, and that makes you smile. Without thinking, you silently mouth the words, "Sweet Caroline, bum, bum, bum..."

Music has the power to turn chaos into calm, transporting you to another time and space. It may also excite and energize you or motivate you during your workout. Conversely, a soothing lullaby will help you gently drift off to sleep.

While musical tastes are personal, the research indicates that certain genres of music are more calming than others. Classical or acoustic playlists may slow your thoughts and ease your heart rate. The slow tempo and predictable rhythm of a song may help synchronize your body's rhythms to a more relaxed state.

If you are feeling disconnected or numb, which often happens with PTSD, listening to more upbeat or energetic music might help stir your emotions and reconnect you with your feelings.

Music's capacity to evoke emotions stems from its ability to stimulate the brain's *limbic system*, which is responsible for emotion and memory processing.

Because musical tastes vary, there are no one-size-fits-all prescriptive playlists to serve as therapeutic listening selections for complex PTSD. Therefore, you get to experiment!

Creating personal playlists that cater to your different emotional needs is a highly effective strategy for mood regulation.

Why not give it a try?

1. Start by identifying the emotions you'd like to manage more effectively.
2. Be as specific as you can: fear, anxiety, sadness, rage, detachment...
3. Experiment with different genres and types of music.
4. Make a note of which ones elicit the desired emotional response.

Example: Whenever I am angry and want to change my state, or when I am grumpy because I must clean the house, I crank up the 80s girl bands.

How can anyone be angry or grumpy when singing along to *The Bangles*, *Bananarama*, *Madonna*, or *Cindy Lauper*? Not me, that is for sure! I'm dancing around the living room with the vacuum cleaner while singing into the feather duster! This era of music makes me feel carefree and happy because it reminds me of a time when I truly was carefree and happy.

The process of creating your own playlists is a therapeutic exercise. It encourages you to engage actively with your emotional landscape, recognize and validate your feelings, and take proactive steps in managing them.

Music engagement promotes a sense of control over your emotional well-being, a valuable asset when navigating the often-unpredictable terrain of PTSD.

Beyond listening to music, engaging in active music-making also has meaningful therapeutic benefits, especially in processing emotions and fostering connections.

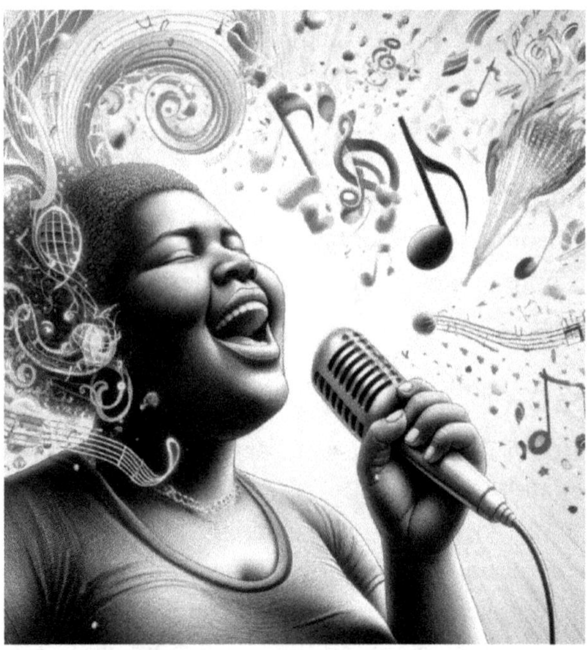

- ✓ **Singing is incredibly cathartic, allowing the expression of emotions that might be hard to articulate in words.**

Singing releases *endorphins*, your body's natural feel-good chemicals. Endorphins alleviate pain and boost mood.

Singing, especially in a group, such as a choir or informal gathering, enhances a sense of community and belonging, counteracting the isolation that often accompanies PTSD.

Playing an instrument offers similar benefits. It provides a focus, a point of concentration that helps distract from distressing thoughts. The physical engagement of playing an instrument—whether it's strumming a guitar, playing a piano, or even beating a drum—can help anchor you in the present moment, providing a break from the often-overwhelming emotions associated with trauma.

Do you play an instrument? No? Well, that's okay, because *learning* to play fosters feelings of achievement and self-efficacy. This is confidence boosting and provides a positive focus in your life. Plus, everyone around the campfire loves the person playing the guitar. I know I do.

Working with a Professional Music Therapist

Music therapy represents a formalized approach to using music for emotional and psychological healing.

Professional music therapists are trained to use music interventions to help clients achieve various therapeutic goals in a clinical and evidence-based practice.

In the context of PTSD, these goals might include managing stress, improving mood, and addressing trauma-related symptoms such as flashbacks and anxiety.

Music therapists work in various settings, including hospitals, clinics, and private practices, and their methods may vary widely depending on the client's needs. They might use active techniques, like playing instruments or singing, to help a client to express feelings they can't yet put into words.

Alternatively, a music therapist might use receptive techniques, like listening to and discussing music, to help clients reflect on their emotions and experiences. The therapeutic relationship is central to this process, providing a safe and supportive environment where clients explore their emotions and experiences without judgment.

If you are interested in exploring music therapy, it's important to seek a therapist credentialed by the appropriate regulatory bodies, such as the *American Music Therapy Association* in the United States. These professionals are equipped with the skills and knowledge to tailor therapeutic interventions that best support your journey towards healing, helping you navigate the complex emotions and challenges associated with PTSD.

Music therapy offers a unique blend of art and science, providing a creative outlet for expression and a structured approach to emotional healing. Whether through creating personal playlists, engaging in active music-making, or participating in structured music therapy sessions, music offers a powerful tool for healing and transformation.

- ✓ **Music resonates with the deepest parts of our being, healing us from the inside out.**

Photography as a Tool for Mindfulness and Healing

In the kaleidoscope of healing, photography emerges not just as an art form but as a therapeutic tool, offering a unique approach to mindfulness and emotional processing. The camera becomes more than a device—it transforms into a medium of connection, grounding, and expression.

Engaging with photography helps cultivate a practice of present-moment awareness, a skill often eroded by the persistent unease and disconnection experienced in PTSD.

When you look through a lens, the world narrows down to that moment, that frame. Everything else falls away, leaving you with the here and now.

This act of focusing is inherently mindful. It anchors you in the present, pulling your thoughts away from past traumas and future anxieties.

Each click of the shutter captures more than one picture. It captures a moment of focused presence, helping to train your mind to stay in the now. The beauty of this practice lies in its simplicity and accessibility.

Whether you're photographing a sprawling landscape, the bustling city streets, or the quiet details of your living room, the act itself diverts attention from internal distress to external beauty, encouraging a shift in perspective that can be both healing and uplifting.

Imagine using your camera to find and capture instances of beauty and joy in your daily life. This practice, akin to a visual form of gratitude, significantly shifts your focus from pain to appreciation.

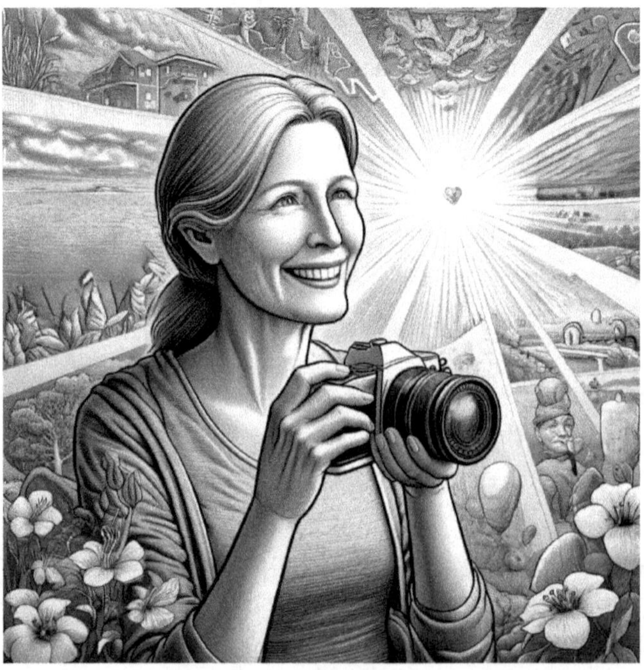

Perhaps you'll capture the morning light streaming through your window, the intricate patterns of a leaf, or a spontaneous smile from a stranger. These captured moments serve as reminders of the beauty and simplicity that life holds, often overlooked in the rush of daily living or the haze of trauma.

Over time, purposefully seeking and acknowledging beauty will foster a more positive outlook, enhancing your capacity to notice and appreciate the good, even on tough days.

Photographic narratives offer another layer of healing potential. By creating photo series that tell a story—your story—you engage in an act of reclaiming and reshaping your narrative. This could involve documenting a typical day, capturing themes of recovery, or articulating through images what words cannot convey.

Selecting what to photograph and what to include in your frame gives you control over how you tell your story. It's a form of self-agency, a way of saying, "This is my perspective, my experience, my truth."

By sharing photo narratives, whether in a personal journal, a blog, or a gallery, you invite understanding and connection. This bridges the gap between your internal experience and the external world.

If you find yourself ready to embark on this photographic journey, remember that the essence of photography, in this context, is not about technical perfection. Instead, it is about expression and connection.

Here are some ideas to get you started:

- Start with whatever camera you have, even if it's just your smartphone.
- Every day, take 10 minutes to snap something that captures your attention.
- Pay attention to lighting.
- Experiment with morning and evening shots.
- Learn perspective by taking photos from different angles.

- ❖ Reflect on how lighting and perspective affect the mood of a photo.
- ❖ Keep it simple.
- ❖ Focus on the process and not the outcome.

Remember, the goal of your photographic journal is to connect with the moment. It is through this connection that you'll find pathways to greater peace and presence.

As you integrate photography into your healing process, let each snapshot be a step toward viewing the world with renewed perspective and hope.

- ✓ **Let the lens bring you closer to the beauty surrounding you that often goes unnoticed. Allow this new awareness to infuse your journey with a lighter, more hopeful stride.**

Dance & Movement: Moving Beyond Trauma

Dance/movement therapy (DMT) offers a wonderful way to connect the movement of your body to the landscape of your emotions. This provides a bridge between physical expression and psychological healing.

Rooted in the principle that mind and body are inseparable, DMT operates on the understanding that changing one will fundamentally affect the other. This form of therapy uses dance and movement to help you engage with your emotions. These emotions are often locked deep inside and not easily accessible through traditional talk therapy.

DMT offers a pathway to express and process emotions through a non-verbal yet extremely articulate medium.

The principles of DMT are centered around the concept of *embodied cognition*. Simply stated: Our bodies hold onto our memories and emotions. We manifest these memories and emotions through posture, movement, and bodily tensions.

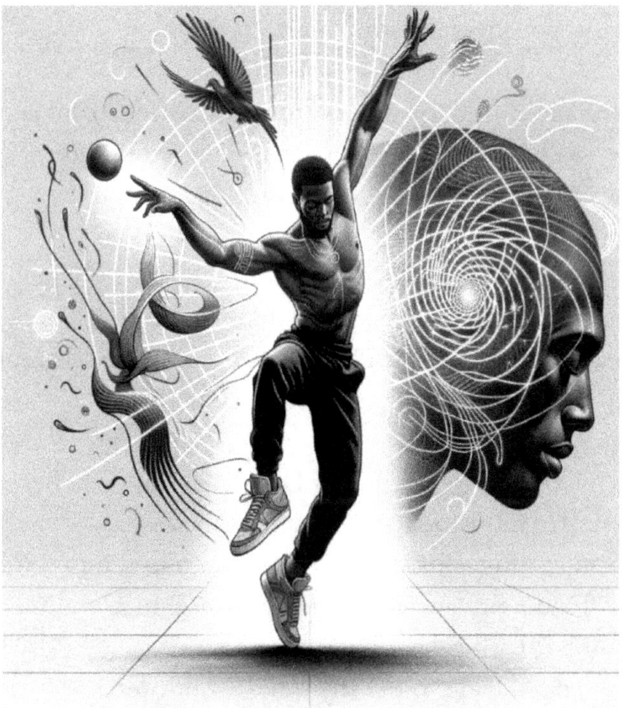

In DMT sessions, therapists guide you through movements that aim to uncover these hidden emotions. This provides a safe space where bodily movements tell their stories. The therapist might ask you to demonstrate your feelings using only your body or to move in ways that explore different emotions.

This practice not only fosters a deeper awareness of how your emotions inhabit your body but also helps to release the emotional energy that might be stuck. This promotes psychological relief and healing.

The awareness of your body and its movements cultivated in DMT can be incredibly uplifting. It allows for a reconnection with parts of yourself that might have been dissociated from your consciousness due to trauma.

This enhanced body awareness improves self-esteem and self-efficacy as you learn to express and manage feelings more effectively.

Additionally, the physical activity involved in DMT helps reduce symptoms of anxiety and depression, which are common companions of PTSD. This is done by releasing endorphins and promoting overall well-being.

If you're considering exploring DMT on your own, here are some simple movements you might start with:

1. Find a private, comfortable space where you feel safe.
2. Start with gentle, intuitive movements.
3. Try swaying to the rhythm of your breath.
4. Stretch your arms out wide.
5. Or curl tightly into a ball, like the *Child's Pose* used in yoga, and rock your body back and forth.
6. Pay attention to how each movement feels and allow your body to guide you.
7. Remember, there is no right or wrong way to move.

This practice helps you become more attuned to your body's needs and emotions. These 7 basic steps are a very brief introduction to more structured DMT exercises; however, these steps may help you decide if DMT is a good fit for your recovery journey.

If you'd like to engage more deeply with DMT, finding a qualified dance/movement therapist is key. Licensed therapists are trained not only in therapeutic techniques but also in movement analysis and dance.

Your DMT therapist will tailor sessions to your specific emotional and physical needs, creating a structured yet flexible environment where you explore your trauma and healing through movement.

When searching for a therapist, consider looking for professionals certified by the *American Dance Therapy Association (ADTA)*. The ADTA ensures the therapist has met rigorous professional standards.

During therapy sessions, expect to focus on creating a harmonious relationship between your body and mind. Your therapist will guide you through movements that resonate with your emotional state, helping you explore and express feelings that might be difficult to articulate verbally.

These sessions often lead to breakthroughs, as the movement may unlock emotions and memories in ways that words cannot.

The therapist's role is to support you through this process, ensuring that the exploration of these sometimes-difficult territories is done safely and therapeutically.

Engaging in DMT provides a dynamic way to navigate the healing process from complex PTSD, offering a form of expression that is both creative and cathartic.

- ✓ **As you move, you not only release the trauma stored in your body but also build a stronger, more resilient self.**

This therapy celebrates the power of movement as a vehicle for emotional expression and personal transformation. It reinforces the idea that through movement, we will indeed move beyond our traumas.

Wrapping it Up

As we close this chapter on creative and expressive therapies, we've traversed the therapeutic landscapes of art, writing, music, photography, and dance.

Each modality offers unique avenues for expression, reflection, and healing, emphasizing the power of creativity in the recovery process.

These therapies provide tools not only to cope with the aftermath of trauma but to transform and transcend it, allowing for a re-engagement of your life in meaningful and joyous ways.

Moving Forward

Looking ahead, the next chapter will explore the role of *Nature and Adventure* therapies in recovering from PTSD.

These therapies extend the therapeutic environment from the confines of a room to the great outdoors, where the natural world provides a backdrop for powerful healing experiences.

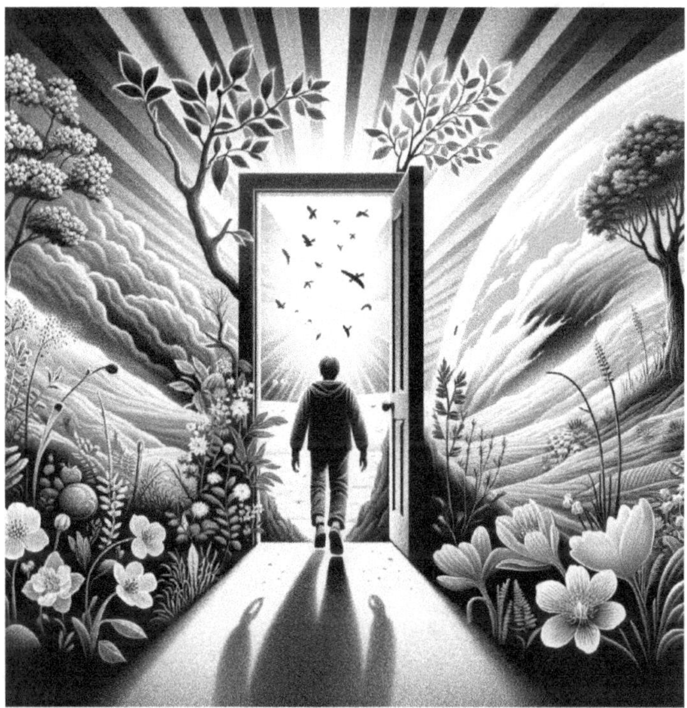

Join me as we step outside, literally and metaphorically, to discover how the earth beneath our feet and the sky above our heads contribute to our journey toward recovery.

Congratulations! You're halfway through this book. Are you finding value in the strategies and information shared?

My goal is to help you feel stronger and more excited to create a pathway for healing of your own design. I hope I'm doing a good job.

Please give this little book a shout out on Amazon.

Why should you review this book?

- It costs nothing & it is a nice thing to do.
- You'll be helping other trauma survivors.
- It takes only a few moments.
- And you'll make me smile.

Use the QR code or follow this link:
https://www.amazon.com/review/B0D91H342T

Your review doesn't need to be long. Just a few sentences will make a big difference!

Here are some ideas for your review:

- What is your favorite part of the book, so far?
- Which strategies or tips do you find helpful?

Thanks for supporting me and being a part of this journey. I value your feedback, and so will others who read it.

Read on and be hopeful!

C.W. Lockhart, PhD

Step 6: Go Outside!

Open the door to step outside. The fresh air greets you like an old friend, a reminder of the world's vastness and your own very special place within it. Nature, with its unscripted beauty and timeless rhythms, offers a unique form of therapy that's both grounding and uplifting.

Embrace the Great Outdoors

For those of us who carry the weight of complex PTSD, particularly those who have served and safeguarded, reconnecting with nature isn't just a leisure activity—it's a vital part of our healing process. The great outdoors provides a stark contrast to the chaotic inner turmoil of PTSD, offering us a wide-open space where our hearts will heal, our minds may rest, and our bodies will rejuvenate.

The Healing Power of Nature: Eco-Therapy Basics

The healing power of nature is well-researched and documented. Studies consistently show that spending time in natural environments combats stress, improves mood, and enhances cognitive functioning. These benefits are particularly vital for individuals dealing with complex PTSD.

Nature's ability to reduce stress is often attributed to its effect on the body's production of stress hormones like cortisol, which are typically elevated whenever we endure chronic stress and anxiety.

Engaging with the natural world via a walk through a forest or a quiet moment in a city park may effectively reduce stress-related hormone levels and foster relaxation and peace.

The sensory-rich environment of nature, the rustling leaves, the softness of grass beneath your feet, and the elaborate patterns of tree bark—may all help improve your mood by providing gentle stimuli for the senses.

This stimulus works by temporarily pulling you away from distressing and intrusive thoughts.

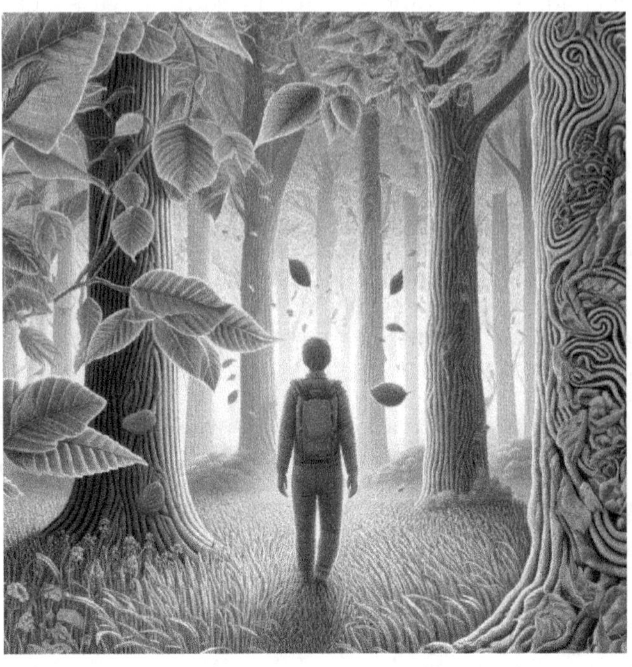

Shades of green and blue, abundant in natural landscapes, are particularly soothing and contribute to feelings of happiness and calmness.

Additionally, bathing in nature enhances cognitive functioning by improving attention and focus, two elements commonly compromised by trauma exposure.

This mental clarity is a balm for the often foggy and fragmented thoughts that accompany complex PTSD.

Simple Ways to Connect with Nature

Connecting with nature doesn't require you to venture far or plan elaborate camping trips into the wilderness.

It can be as simple as tending to a plant in your living room, feeding birds at a local park, or even just opening a window to let natural light and fresh air into your space.

Finding pockets of nature like community gardens, rooftop green spaces, or tree-lined streets offer daily touchpoints with the natural world if you live in an urban area.

If you have access to a balcony or a small yard, consider creating a mini sanctuary with potted plants, a few comfortable chairs, and perhaps a bird feeder to attract local wildlife.

Even small episodic interactions with nature can be woven into your daily routine as micro-doses of eco-therapy without requiring extensive travel or time commitment.

Eco-Therapy Practices

Eco-therapy involves structured practices that use nature to promote mental and emotional well-being. One such practice is forest bathing, or *Shinrin-yoku*, a concept developed in Japan that involves simply being in the presence of trees.

Shinrin-yoku doesn't require hiking or intense physical exercise. Instead, the practice focuses on quietly observing nature and absorbing the forest atmosphere through all your senses. This immersive experience remarkably reduces stress, increases energy, and improves sleep, making it an ideal therapeutic activity for those recovering from PTSD.

Another accessible eco-therapy practice involves nature walks. These walks can be adapted to fit accessibility needs and varying fitness levels. They may be solo or group efforts. These relaxing walks are less about physical exertion and more about mindfulness—paying close attention to the sights, sounds, and smells around you as you move. This mindful engagement helps bring your thoughts into the present and fosters a peaceful mind.

Incorporating Nature into Healing

Integrating regular nature-based activities into your healing journey will transform your relationship with the world around you. Start by scheduling short, regular intervals dedicated to outdoor activities. Even 15 to 30 minutes will be beneficial. Gradually, as you begin to feel the benefits, you might find yourself naturally inclined to increase the time you spend outdoors.

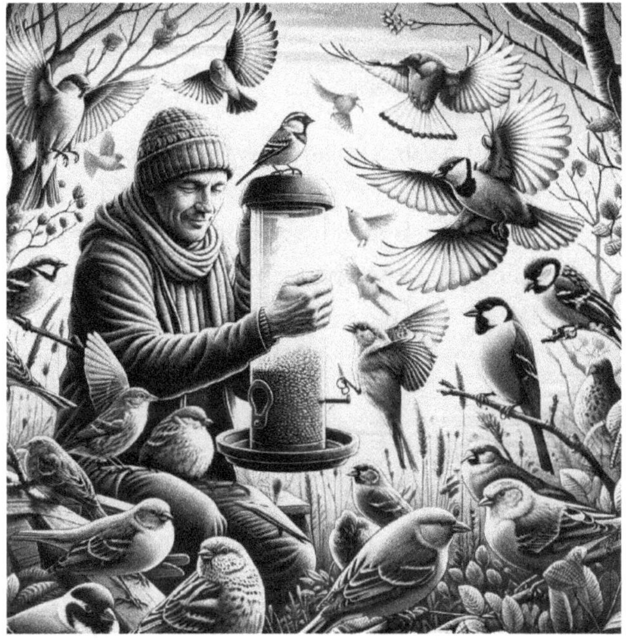

- ✓ **Be intentional about your activities in nature.**

For instance, you could set a goal to identify new birds, plants, or trees on each walk, which adds an element of focus and engagement to your outings.

Alternatively, you could use your nature time for reflection, meditation, or sitting quietly and journaling your experiences and feelings.

Setting an intentional goal before entering your practice helps deepen the therapeutic impact of your time, making it an integral part of your healing strategy.

As you incorporate these practices, remember that your engagement with nature is unique to you and you, alone.

What works for others may not work for you, and that's perfectly okay.

The goal is to find natural settings and activities that resonate with your preferences and therapeutic needs. Strive to create a personalized approach to eco-therapy that supports your individual healing process. Through this tailored engagement, you harness the restorative power of nature, finding not just solace but a deepened source of renewal and strength.

Gardening as a Therapeutic Practice

A humble vegetable garden can be a multipurpose sanctuary, providing a sense of inner peace and a source of healthy foods for your table.

The garden offers a unique space for restoration and growth. The simple acts of planting seeds, watering, tending, weeding, and harvesting may be deeply therapeutic and considerably enhance both your physical and mental well-being.

Nurturing plants for food or simple beauty provides a wonderful sense of accomplishment and a connection to Earth. It's all about cultivating your own sense of peace and stability.

The cyclical nature of gardening tasks rotates with the seasons, keeping you grounded in time and space. This connection between the changing seasons and the ongoing needs of your plants helps keep you anchored in the now while still looking toward the future.

- ✓ **In the garden, every seed planted is a tiny symbol of hope, a physical manifestation of your capacity to influence your environment in positive ways.**

Watching something grow from a seed to a plant under your care is incredibly rewarding and significantly boosts your self-esteem and sense of efficacy. These feelings are especially beneficial to offset the times when you feel powerless or disconnected.

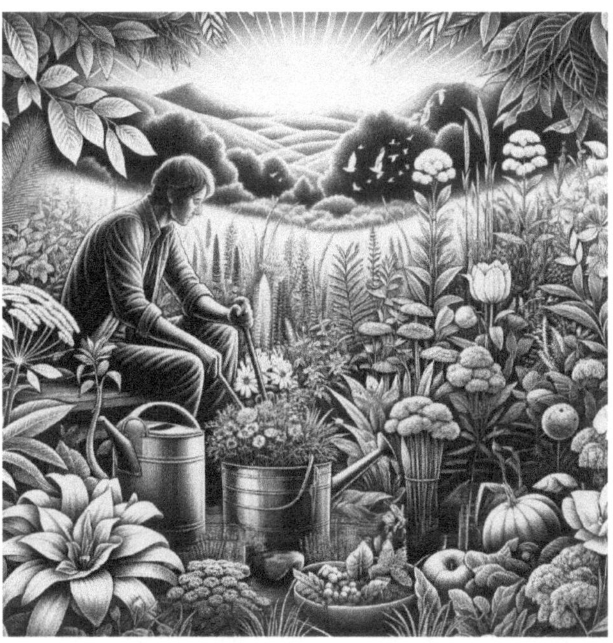

Start a Healing Garden

You can create a healing garden of your own. Starting your garden does not require a vast space or expert-level skills. Start very small, with perhaps just a few containers on a balcony or stoop.

If you'd like to garden on a larger scale but do not have access to space, ask around your neighborhood. Perhaps there is an available plot in a community garden.

- ✓ **Community gardening is a beautiful way to build connections, socialize, learn from other gardeners, and foster a sense of camaraderie.**

As with other recovery modalities presented in the previous chapters, the key is to focus on the process rather than the outcome.

Here are some tips to get you started:

1. Choose plants compatible with local temperatures.
2. Herbs, like mint and rosemary, are low maintenance and useful in your kitchen.
3. Vegetables thrive in small garden beds or larger containers.
4. When setting up your space, consider accessibility and comfort.
5. Raised beds or elevated containers make gardening more manageable.
6. Select simple, easy-to-use tools, like a handheld trowel and spade.
7. Keep pathways clear and easy to navigate.
8. Cultivating a low-stress experience will encourage you to engage regularly.

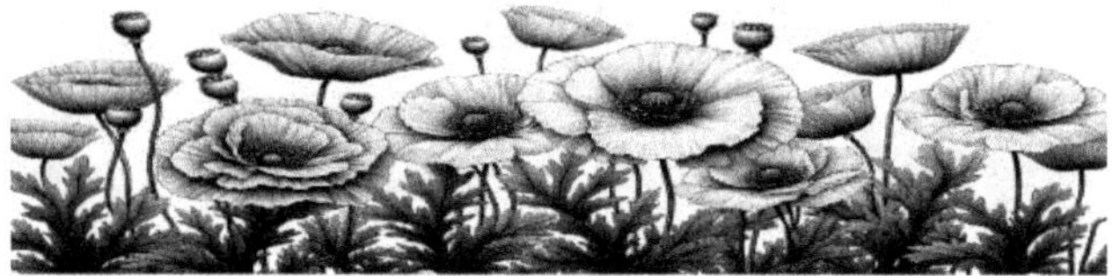

The Solace of Water

Swimming for Recovery

Like other forms of cardio exercise, swimming emerges as a powerful therapeutic tool for individuals grappling with PTSD. The physicality of swimming requires a focus that will help pull your thoughts away from distressing patterns, centering you in the rhythm of your strokes and breaths.

This meditative aspect of swimming greatly reduces stress levels. The repetitive motions and controlled breathing inherent in swimming mimic relaxation techniques used in both meditation and yoga.

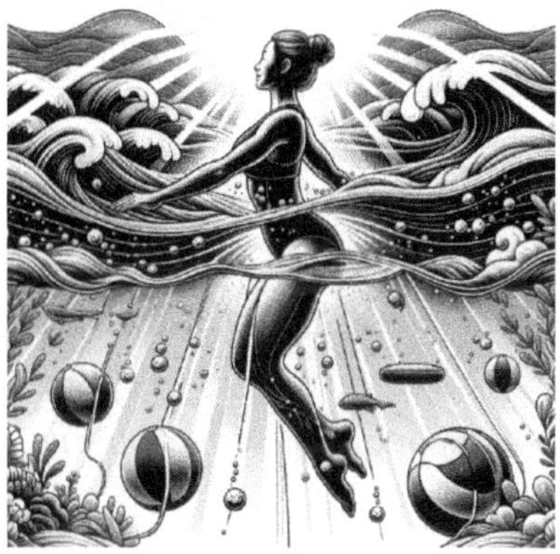

The buoyancy of water provides a unique form of resistance that is both gentle and supportive, allowing for physical exercise without the strain on joints and muscles that land-based workouts might invoke.

Regular engagement in open-water or pool swimming improves mood and enhances physical health.

- ✓ **The physical exercise involved in swimming stimulates the release of endorphins, the body's natural mood lifters.**

Endorphins combat the feelings of depression and anxiety that often accompany PTSD. Additionally, the aerobic nature of swimming improves cardiovascular health and increases overall energy levels.

Aquatic Therapy

Taking the therapeutic benefits of water one step further, aquatic therapy involves structured activities and exercises performed in a water-based environment, typically under the guidance of a trained therapist.

This form of therapy combines the soothing properties of water with specific therapeutic exercises designed to address the physical and emotional aspects of injury and trauma.

Aquatic therapy sessions might include guided movements, floating exercises, or even gentle water-based games designed to reduce muscle tension, improve emotional regulation, and enhance self-esteem.

The controlled environment of aquatic therapy ensures safety and comfort, allowing you to explore physical movements that might be challenging on land. Buoyancy reduces the impact on the body, making it easier to perform exercises to improve flexibility, strength, and endurance. Warm, therapeutic pools help relax muscles and increase blood circulation, further aiding in the healing process. This supportive setting of aqua therapy allows for a gradual building of physical capabilities, which significantly boosts self-confidence. These are important steps in reclaiming your body's strength, post-trauma.

Creating Water Rituals

Incorporating water into your daily routine is a simple yet effective way to harness therapeutic benefits. Creating your own rituals will provide regular moments of calm and reflection in your day.

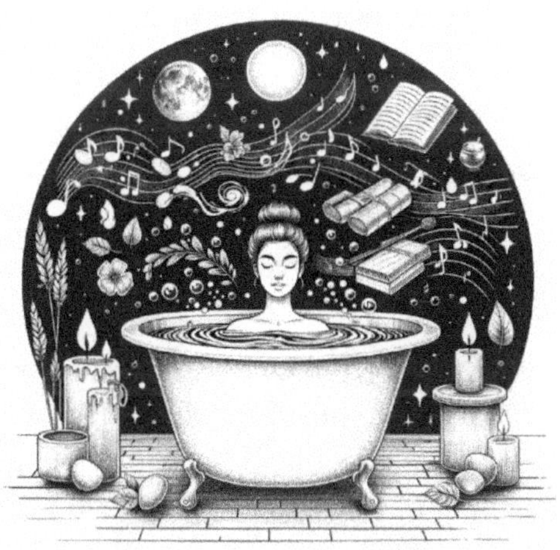

These rituals can be as simple as taking an extra-long shower, allowing the warmth and sound of the water to soothe you. Another accessible and relaxing water ritual is bathing.

Bath water infused with calming substances like Epsom salts or essential oils may be quite therapeutic. Combining warm water and these additives helps reduce physical tension, soothe your skin, and promote deep relaxation.

You may enhance your ritual by adding other elements, like soft music, dim lighting, or candles, to create a spa-like atmosphere that encourages deep relaxation. When integrated into your routine, these water rituals will serve as daily touchstones of calm, helping to manage stress and enhance your overall sense of well-being.

Adventure Therapy: Finding Healing in Adrenaline

Adventure therapy offers a dynamic and exhilarating approach to healing that blends the thrill of outdoor activities with the therapeutic process of overcoming personal challenges. This form of therapy harnesses activities such as rock climbing, white-water rafting, or zip-lining, which not only push your physical limits but also challenge your emotional and psychological resilience.

Engaging in adventurous pursuits provides a unique opportunity to confront your fears, develop trust in yourself and others, and experience the joy of achievement. For someone navigating the complexities of PTSD, the controlled, supportive environment of adventure therapy might be particularly beneficial, offering a space to explore your strengths and vulnerabilities in new and empowering ways.

One of the core principles of adventure therapy is the concept of managed risk. Unlike the uncontrollable risks that may have characterized your traumatic experiences, the risks in adventure therapy are calculated and carefully monitored by trained professionals.

This controlled risk-setting provides a safe space to face your fears and challenges without feeling overwhelmed. For example, when you climb a rock wall, you are harnessed and guided by experienced instructors who ensure your safety while encouraging you to push your boundaries. This setup allows you to experience both the fear of climbing higher and the support that makes it safe to do so.

Overcoming fears boosts your self-efficacy—your belief in your ability to handle challenges—and resilience, reinforcing a sense of competence and strength that is transformative.

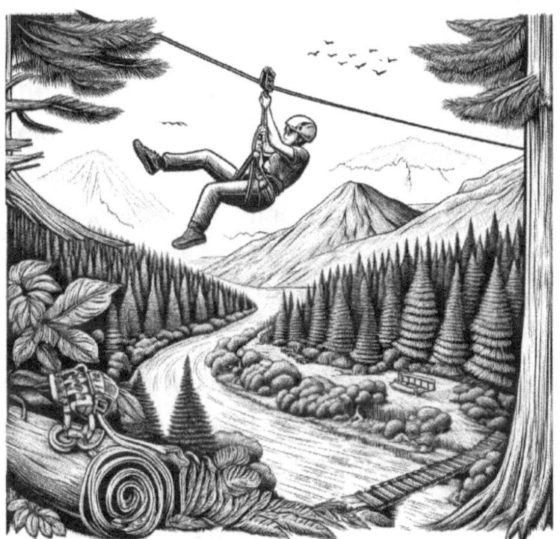

If you are new to adventure therapy or outdoor activities, starting with accessible adventures is key. Choose activities that match your current physical and emotional readiness.

Many adventure therapy programs offer a range of activities tailored to different skill levels and therapeutic needs. These activities prioritize your emotional comfort and gradual progress, ensuring the adventure remains therapeutic rather than overwhelming.

Finding Adventure Therapy Programs

Locating reputable adventure therapy programs that align with your needs will greatly influence your healing experience. When searching for a program, consider what aspects of your PTSD you hope to address and what types of activities you're interested in.

Many programs offer tailored sessions focused on building trust, improving communication, or enhancing self-esteem. It's also important to check the credentials of the program providers. Look for programs led by certified therapists or professionals with specialized training in both adventure activities and psychological therapy. These qualifications indicate that the providers are trained and equipped to handle your physical safety and emotional well-being.

Once you find a program that resonates with you, setting clear expectations for your participation helps optimize your experience. Most reputable programs offer an initial assessment or consultation to discuss your goals, concerns, and any limitations you might have. Use this opportunity to ask about the structure of the sessions, the safety measures in place, and the therapeutic approaches used. Understanding these elements will help you feel more prepared and secure.

Participating in adventure therapy is a significant step forward in your recovery from complex PTSD. It offers a blend of physical challenges and therapeutic insights that catalyze personal growth and healing.

As you climb a rock face, paddle through rapids, strap on a scuba tank, or soar down a zip line, you're engaging in thrilling physical activities and embarking on a psychological adventure. Each challenge you overcome in the safe, supportive environment reinforces your capacity to navigate the complexities of your trauma and recovery.

With each step, paddle, and climb, you achieve more than simply moving through the landscape. You are moving forward in your healing process and embracing the risks and rewards of a fuller, more resilient life.

Hiking and Pilgrimage for Emotional Resilience

Lace up your hiking boots and set out on a trail. Notice how the rhythm of your steps becomes a meditative practice, grounding you in the moment. Each step carries you not just across the physical terrain but deeper into your own internal landscape to a place where the distant echoes of past traumas may be explored and understood within the context of the expansive natural world around you.

The act of hiking, especially on longer or more difficult trails, mirrors the emotional resilience and endurance required to navigate complex PTSD. The journey is long and sometimes very hard, but each step forward is a step toward healing, a testament to your strength and resolve.

The physical challenge of hiking, with its ups and downs, reflects the mental and emotional challenges you face. Overcoming a steep climb or navigating a tricky trail section will boost your confidence, reinforcing your ability to tackle difficult tasks and overcome obstacles in other areas of your life.

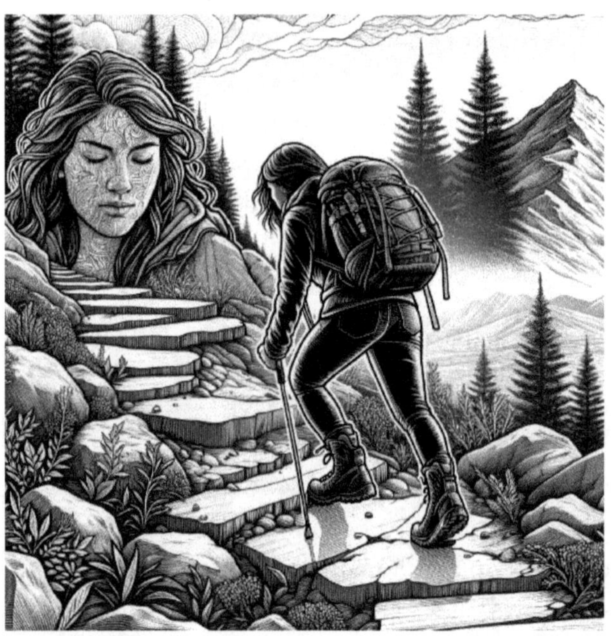

An intrinsic benefit of hiking and long-distance walking is the constant connection with nature. This connection with the outside world intensifies the physicality, providing a backdrop of serene landscapes and the tranquil sounds of the wilderness, which have a naturally soothing effect on the mind. This connection deepens your sense of being part of something much larger than yourself, which is a valuable perspective when dealing with personal trauma.

Hiking and long-distant walking provide both physical and emotional release. Walking a pilgrimage takes this process one step further by engaging your mind, body, and spirit in a journey of recovery and discovery.

A Story of Transformation

In 2014, as a rather unlikely pilgrim, I embarked on my first pilgrimage. Armed only with my humor and a healthy dose of grit, I struck out on a quest to recover and reclaim my life. The path I would follow was along the ancient pilgrimage route known as the *Camino de Santiago* in western Spain.

Several months before leaving for my trip, I had never even heard of the Camino de Santiago and didn't know anyone who had ever walked a pilgrimage. But one night, while binge-watching *Netflix*, as was my norm back then, I stumbled across *The Way*, a movie starring Martin Sheen. My reaction to the film put everything in motion.

After the movie, I asked my boys, "Do you think I could walk 500 miles?" They shook their heads and laughed. So, the next day, I drove to my favorite outdoor store, *REI*, and bought a backpack and a new pair of boots. Game on!

I started my training right away. At first, it was just a short walk down to the mailbox and back. And then a short walk soon became a mile. Little by little, with heaps of self-compassion and a degree of gentleness I had never reserved for myself, I worked up to twelve miles per day. I was ready! Well, at least I thought so.

The physical transformation had been nearly instantaneous. From the moment I decided to leave the sofa to the day I walked my first 12-miler, I could measure the results. My efforts were marked with constant progress, progress that I could quantify and track.

Of course, one of the first things I noticed registered on the bathroom scale. I was losing weight. My cardio was improving. It no longer killed me to walk up the steep drive to my house after fetching the mail. My arms, legs, and torso were firming up. I was still a far cry from that boot camp body of my youth, way back when I was *harder than a woodpecker's lips*. But I couldn't dispute the progress.

I thought that walking every day in the great outdoors would be my cure. And in part, it was. But I had a long way to go.

When I got off the plane in Madrid, all alone, panic set in. *What in the hell was I thinking?* For longer than I care to admit, I hid out in the ladies' bathroom, too frightened to face the bustling airport and connect to the next leg of my journey, a train ride to Pamplona.

I hid so long that I missed the last train. I was stuck in Madrid. Back then, I didn't use public transportation. I just couldn't. So, *I adjusted fire* and came up with another plan.

After a quick and relatively painless engagement at the rental car counter, I was on the road to Pamplona.

Of course, my struggles with C-PTSD didn't end when I dropped off the car. No. I was in for a whole month of adventure. Days were chock-full of physical and emotional obstacles, forcing me from my comfort zone. There was nothing to do about it but face my fears. And I did, in small and huge ways every day.

For me, pilgrimage is so very transformative. Walking is my medicine of choice, and giving myself the wide-open space and time to reflect is my favorite self-talk therapy. I love it so much that I wrote a book about my first experience.

Blanket of Stars: Thru-Hiking the Camino de Santiago was born of gratitude and a sincere hope my experiences might help others. So far, the feedback has been wonderfully uplifting. I have met and corresponded with handfuls of unlikely pilgrims who picked up my book on a whim and headed to their favorite outdoor stores to make pilgrimage their new realities.

For the past decade, I have embarked on a pilgrimage each year. I've now walked along the Camino eight times. I completed a long section of the *Via Francigena* in Italy, walking from Lucca to Rome. I have also traversed 1200 kilometers around a Japanese island, walking a Buddhist pilgrimage. This trail changed my worldview in countless positive ways.

As you've probably guessed, I wrote a book about that one, too: *Walking with Buddha: Pilgrimage on the Shikoku 88-temple trail.*

So, what has a decade of pilgrimage taught me? At the risk of sounding hyperbolic, pilgrimage has taught me *everything.* More accurately, pilgrimage has *rewired* my brain. It has flushed out years of gunk and re-taught me everything—or at least everything I need to know about love, hope, faith, recovery, and living my best life.

The camaraderie and energy of pilgrimage hiking are addictive. In my quest to heal and live a life of my design, I have met many brothers and sisters-in-arms. Veterans from all over the world gravitate to these ancient paths with similar goals and determinations.

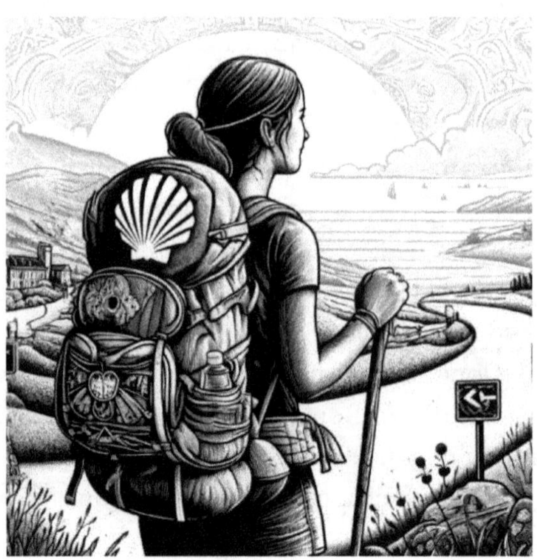

My story and the stories shared by others underscore the transformative power of taking a long hike or walking a pilgrimage. These inspirational stories reveal pathways to emotional resilience and physical well-being, where the act of way-making is a metaphor for moving forward with recovery.

While each person's story is unique and deeply personal, pilgrimage stories share common elements like self-compassion, forgiveness, hope, higher self-esteem, better health, and enhanced abilities to cope with past traumas.

Planning a Personal Pilgrimage or Hiking Journey

Embarking on a personal pilgrimage or a hiking journey requires thoughtful preparation, both logistically and emotionally. Start by setting clear intentions for your hike.

Ask yourself what you hope to achieve or explore during this time. Are you looking to find peace, seek answers, or simply give yourself space to grieve?

Understanding your motivations will guide your choices in planning the route, the duration, and the pace of your hike. The importance of selecting a destination that resonates with you personally cannot be overstated. It could be a place with a special meaning, a landscape that inspires you, or a path that challenges you.

- ✓ **When planning, consider not just the physical demands of the hike but also the emotional implications.**

A journey that's too physically demanding might damage your emotional resilience, while an overly familiar path might not provide the challenge needed for meaningful engagement.

Gather detailed information about the trail. Conduct online searches, peruse guidebooks, and watch a few YouTube videos.

The information is out there, and gathering it is part of the fun.

Your advanced preparation will not only ensure a smoother experience but also help to ease anxiety.

This will allow you more mental energy to focus on the deeper emotional and spiritual aspects of your journey.

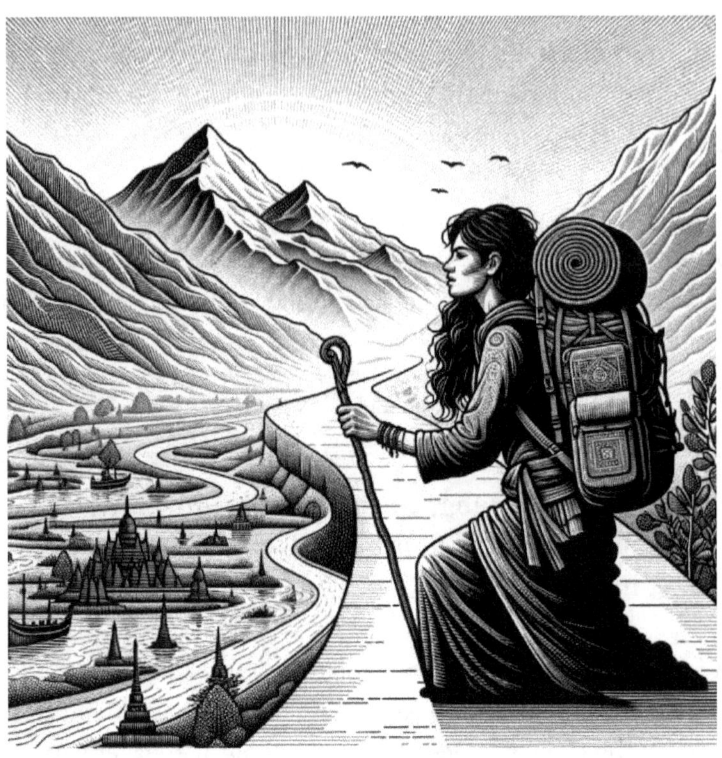

Safety and Preparedness

Safety is paramount when undertaking any outdoor activity, and hiking or making a pilgrimage are no exceptions. Take an inventory of your physical and emotional preparedness.

Physically, ensure you have the right gear, including appropriate footwear, clothing, and a well-packed backpack with essentials like a first aid kit. Educate yourself about the terrain, potential weather changes, and any wildlife you might encounter.

Emotionally, it's important to prepare for the solitude and introspection that often comes with a long hike. This might involve setting up a support system before you leave, such as scheduled check-ins with a friend or therapist.

Be prepared for the emotional ups and downs that may arise. Bringing along a journal to write down your thoughts and feelings will be a helpful way to process emotions as you go.

Additionally, practicing mindfulness and grounding techniques will help manage emotional distress that might surface on the trail.

Hiking and walking pilgrimages offer a unique blend of physical challenge and emotional engagement, making them powerful tools for building resilience and fostering healing.

As you walk, let each step remind you of your strength, endurance, and capacity to move forward, no matter how difficult the path may seem.

Wrapping it up

As we conclude this exploration of nature and adventure therapies, we've discovered that participating in the natural world will play an invaluable role in our healing processes.

Big or small, wildly adventurous or mild, each modality presented offers unique benefits that can be tailored to support your journey toward recovery.

Moving Forward

Our next chapter will explore community and support systems. We will explore how connecting with others, sharing experiences, and building relationships provides strength and comfort as we continue our paths of recovery.

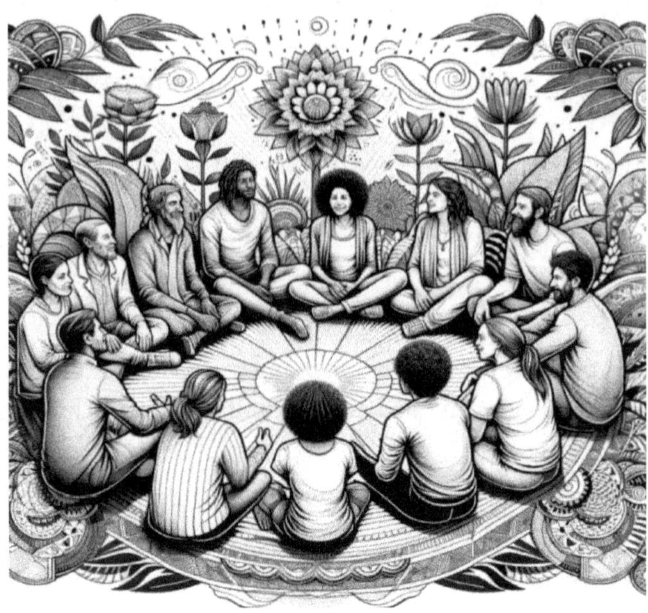

Step 7: Build a Supportive Lifestyle

Structure your day for success. Routine gets a bad rap. We sometimes view it as monotonous or stifling. However, for someone managing complex PTSD, especially if you have served in the military, routine can be a sanctuary.

Routine offers a sense of predictability in a world that often feels frighteningly unpredictable. Establishing a consistent daily routine helps reduce anxiety by minimizing the number of decisions you need to make about basic daily activities.

When your brain knows *what* to expect, it can use less energy worrying about *what comes next.* The comfort of routine lies in its familiarity.

Its rhythm guides your days, offering a gentle structure that makes the world seem a little less chaotic.

A routine conducive to healing might start with a morning ritual, perhaps a cup of tea followed by a few minutes of stretching or meditation to ground yourself for the day.

Integrating such self-care practices early into your daily routine will mitigate the symptoms of PTSD, providing regular touchpoints that remind you to focus on the present.

Regularly scheduled therapy sessions and planned social interactions also form part of this routine and ensure you consistently work toward recovery in a structured way.

Time Management Tips

Managing your time effectively is imperative to maintaining a routine that effectively supports your recovery goals. Prioritization is key here. It's important to distinguish between what must be done and what can wait.

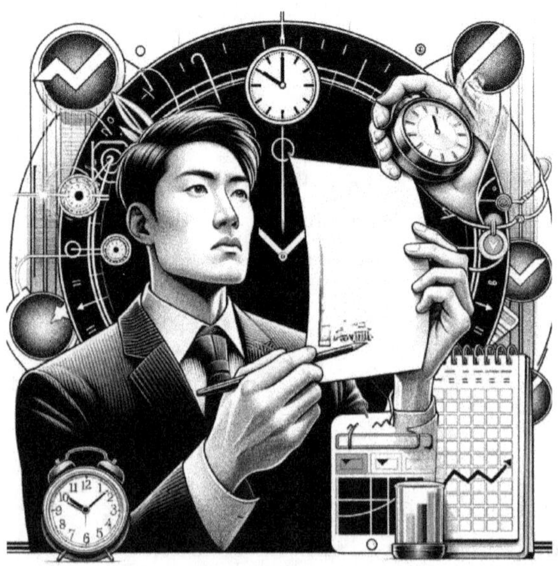

Start by identifying activities that directly contribute to your well-being—therapy appointments, medication times, personal hygiene, meals, physical exercise, and sleep.

- ✓ **Treat these as non-negotiable parts of your day.**

To help manage your time, consider using tools like planners or digital calendars, where you visually map out your day. This helps you allocate time blocks for specific activities, reducing the risk of scheduling conflicts and ensuring adequate time for self-care.

Set reminders! On the road to recovery, so many things are calling out for your attention. It can all be overwhelming, making it easy to forget an appointment or meet up with friends or a loved one. Setting reminders will help you stay on track and manage your commitments.

Incorporating Flexibility

While a routine provides structure, it's essential to build in flexibility to accommodate the ebb and flow of PTSD symptoms, which vary in intensity from day to day.

On days when symptoms are more pronounced, you might need to adjust your routine to include more self-care or reschedule activities that require substantial mental or physical energy.

- ✓ **Allowing yourself flexibility helps you maintain a routine without feeling pressured or overwhelmed.**

It's helpful to have a *Plan B* for days when sticking to your usual routine isn't feasible. This might include simpler or shorter versions of planned activities, like doing a 10-minute meditation instead of a 30-minute one or walking around the block instead of going for a longer run.

By planning for these adjustments, you ensure that you still have a structure for your day but one that respects your current needs and limits.

Nutritional Strategies to Support Mental Health

The Gut-Brain Connection

It's often said, somewhat whimsically, that the stomach is a second brain. This isn't just a poetic metaphor but a reflection of the powerful connection between your gut health and your mental well-being, a link that's especially significant when you're managing complex PTSD.

Emerging research has illuminated how the gut and brain communicate via the vagus nerve and various biochemical pathways, including neurotransmitters and hormones. This bidirectional communication system means that digestive health influences brain function and, consequently, mood and stress levels.

For those of us dealing with PTSD, understanding this connection is nothing short of life-altering. The gut produces about 95% of serotonin, a neurotransmitter that helps regulate mood, appetite, and sleep—three areas that are particularly disrupted by PTSD.

An imbalance in your gut flora leads to a decrease in serotonin production, which might exacerbate anxiety and depression symptoms. Therefore, nurturing your gut health through diet becomes not just about physical health.

- ✓ **Diet is integral to managing your mental health.**

Foods to Embrace and Avoid

Navigating the world of nutrition can be overwhelming for anyone. Let's simplify it by focusing on what to embrace and what to avoid.

Foods rich in probiotics, like yogurt, kefir, and fermented foods such as sauerkraut and kimchi, help to maintain a healthy gut flora, potentially improving your mood and emotional health.

Fiber-rich foods like fruits, vegetables, and whole grains are also vital as they promote the growth of beneficial gut bacteria.

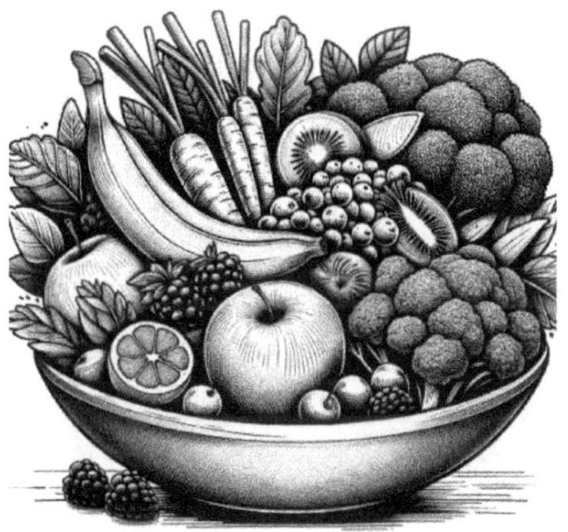

On the other hand, certain foods might do more harm than good when it comes to managing PTSD symptoms.

High levels of caffeine can provoke anxiety and disrupt sleep patterns, while a high intake of sugar may lead to fluctuations in blood sugar levels, which increases mood swings and irritability.

Processed foods, often high in sugar and fat, alter the balance of your gut bacteria and exacerbate inflammation, which is already linked to several mental health issues.

By increasing your intake of gut-friendly foods and reducing your intake of foods that potentially exasperate your PTSD symptoms, you'll make great strides in stabilizing your mood and improving your overall well-being.

The role nutrition plays in our physical and mental health cannot simply be addressed in a few paragraphs, a chapter, or even an entire book. I encourage you to continue your research about this vital link.

The information is out there, so much so that the plethora of research and opinions can drag you down into an endless rabbit hole. So, I recommend sampling it only. Treat it like a buffet jam-packed with a myriad of humble and exotic dishes and everything in between. Take only what you need and leave the rest.

Hydration and Mental Health

Hydration plays a vital role in maintaining your mental health. This fact is often overlooked. Dehydration leads to increased cortisol levels, the stress hormone that is frequently elevated with PTSD.

Dehydration makes managing stress and anxiety more challenging. Additionally, proper hydration is critical for the optimal function of serotonin and other neurotransmitters that regulate mood and anxiety.

- ✓ **Drink at least eight glasses of water a day.**

Drinking eight glasses of water every day is old news, but it is a good benchmark. Of course, personal needs vary based on factors like activity level and climate.

Remember, beverages like caffeinated drinks and alcohol may dehydrate you, so remember to balance these with plenty of water throughout the day.

If you find it challenging to drink your daily water goal, try incorporating foods with high water content. Cucumbers, celery, watermelon, and oranges are all great examples of high-water content foods.

Simple Changes

Start small. Implementing nutritional and water intake changes doesn't have to be an all-or-nothing approach, especially when considering the unique set of challenges you are already living with.

Begin by introducing one probiotic-rich food into your diet each week or swapping out your afternoon coffee for water or an herbal tea. These minor adjustments, over time, will make a major difference.

- ✓ **Budget and accessibility undoubtably affect our abilities to make dietary changes.**

Trust me, I've endured more bowls of ramen and easy mac & cheese than I care to recall. And if that is where you are, I totally get it. But we can start small.

- ✓ **Take control of what you can. And reach out for help.**

Community resources such as local food banks or community gardens can be invaluable in accessing healthy food options.

Additionally, planning your weekly meals will help manage your budget and nutritional intake. Prepping ensures you have all the necessary ingredients to make healthy meals without the stress of last-minute decisions.

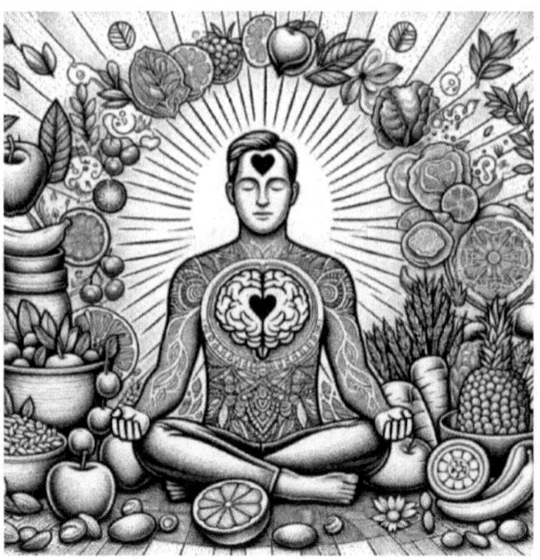

By gradually incorporating these strategies into your daily life, you create a supportive nutritional foundation that not only bolsters your physical health but is also pivotal in managing your mental health.

This holistic approach to wellness is key in the management of PTSD, where every positive change improves your overall quality of life.

The Importance of Sleep in PTSD Recovery

Sleep is essential but often elusive. We need it for our bodies and minds to repair and rejuvenate, but for many of us, our nights often become battlegrounds. This disruption not only leaves us exhausted but also perpetuates the cycle of symptoms.

Poor sleep exacerbates anxiety, depression, and stress. Understanding and addressing these sleep disturbances is, therefore, not just about getting enough rest but about breaking a cycle of disruption that hinders your overall recovery and well-being.

Sleep disturbances in PTSD manifest in various forms, including difficulty falling asleep, staying asleep, or experiencing restorative sleep.

The hyperarousal state associated with PTSD means your body is constantly on alert, scanning for threats, making it difficult to relax enough to fall sleep.

Hyperarousal can be triggered by seemingly innocuous nighttime noises or even by absolute silence. An overly vigilant mind might interpret silence as a sign of impending danger. The irony is palpable. The darkness meant to cloak you in rest only heightens your sense of vulnerability.

Creating a calming bedtime routine is a transformative strategy. This routine serves as a signal to your body and mind that it is time to wind down and shift from a state of alertness to one of relaxation.

Set a consistent bedtime and wake-up time. This will help regulate your internal clock.

About an hour before sleep, engage in relaxing activities. Try reading a book, listening to gentle music, or practicing relaxation exercises like deep breathing or progressive muscle relaxation. These activities help decrease your heart rate and lower your stress levels, making it easier to fall asleep.

Optimize your sleep environment to combat sleep disturbances. Your bedroom should be a sanctuary that promotes relaxation. Consider the comfort of your mattress and pillows, the light levels, and the temperature. These are all factors that influence sleep quality.

Reducing blue light exposure from screens before bedtime is necessary. Blue light is known to interfere with melatonin production, the hormone responsible for regulating sleep.

Blackout curtains or a sleep mask help manage light exposure, and white noise machines or apps provide a soothing backdrop that masks disruptive sounds.

Dealing with nightmares and night terrors is particularly challenging. But these disturbances are also manageable with the right strategies.

One approach is *Image Rehearsal Therapy* (IRT), a cognitive-behavioral technique where you rewrite the ending of your nightmares while awake, making them less threatening. You then mentally rehearse these new versions before sleeping. This helps reduce the frequency and intensity of nightmares.

Keeping a dream journal may also be helpful. This allows you to record and identify themes or triggers within your nightmares. Once Identified, these themes and triggers can be further explored and addressed in therapy.

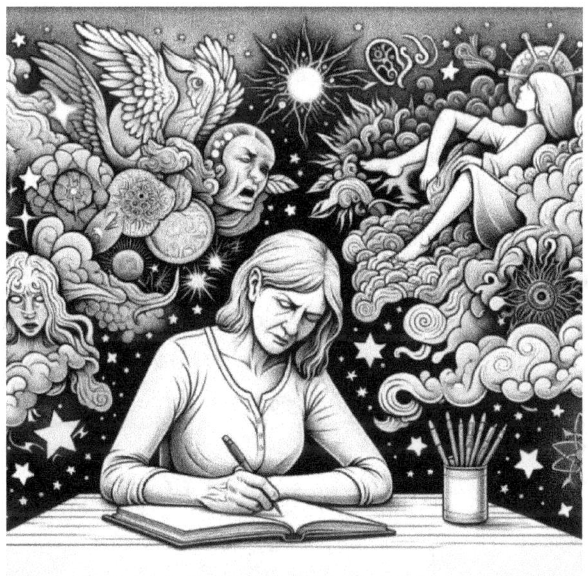

For those struggling with severe sleep disturbances, professional help can be invaluable. *Cognitive Behavioral Therapy for Insomnia* (CBT-I) is an effective treatment that addresses the thoughts and behaviors that prevent you from sleeping well.

Techniques like stimulus control help reinforce the bed as a cue for sleep rather than wakefulness. Sleep restriction, which limits the time spent in bed, increases sleep efficiency.

Consulting with a healthcare provider trained in these therapies will provide you with a tailored approach to improving your sleep while considering the specific challenges posed by C-PTSD.

Incorporating sleep strategies into your life does not mean that every night will be perfect. Instead, strategies provide a framework to substantially improve your ability to get the restful sleep needed. This, in turn, helps reduce the intensity of PTSD symptoms during the day, creating a beneficial cycle of better days and better nights, and in turn, propels you forward in your recovery.

Embracing any type of change requires patience and persistence. Altering sleep habits will take time. However, the benefits to your mental and physical health are noteworthy. This makes every effort worthwhile as you work towards reclaiming the night and the peace it is meant to bring.

Creating a Safe and Healing Home Environment

Your home should be your sanctuary, a place where you can retreat and rejuvenate. The impact of a healing environment cannot be overstated—it becomes a pivotal foundation in our recovery journey.

The spaces we inhabit deeply influence our feelings of safety and calm, reflecting and affecting our inner state. When your living space is organized, serene, and reflective of your personal tastes, it remarkably reduces anxiety and helps manage PTSD symptoms more effectively. Conversely, a chaotic or distressing space may trigger anxiety and make it difficult to find peace or comfort.

Let's start by considering the importance of decluttering. Clutter is more than just physical stuff—it serves as a visual representation of mental chaos.

It's all too easy for your surroundings to become cluttered with items that hold no purpose or joy, and this subconsciously echoes the turmoil within, making it harder to find peace.

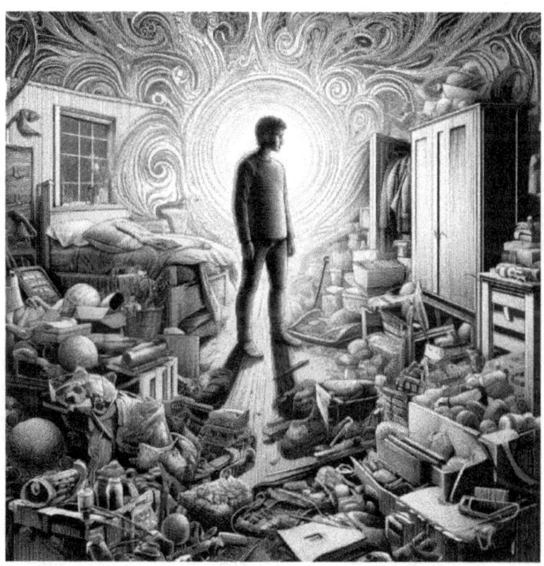

✓ **Begin by decluttering your living spaces.**

This doesn't mean you have to live minimally. Instead, everything you choose to keep around you should serve a purpose, whether it's functional or simply brings you joy. Decluttering is therapeutic, symbolizing the shedding of unnecessary burdens and simplifying your environment to better support your mental health.

Incorporating elements of nature into your home also plays a transformative role in creating a healing atmosphere. Studies have shown that being around elements like plants, water, or even views of the outdoors can lower blood pressure, reduce stress, and enhance overall well-being.

You might start by integrating easy-to-care-for indoor plants. A plant not only beautifies your space but also improves air quality and brings a sense of life and growth into your home.

If you enjoy the sound of water, consider a small indoor fountain. The sound of flowing water may be incredibly soothing and serve as a continuous reminder to flow with the experiences of life. Accept and let go, much like water does.

Creating personal spaces within your home that cater to relaxation and self-care is essential. Designate a specific area as your tranquil corner—perhaps a cozy spot by the window with a comfortable chair and soft lighting where you read, meditate, or simply sit and breathe.

A dedicated space for relaxation acts as a physical boundary within your home, signaling to your mind that entering this space means entering a state of calm and comfort.

Over time, just being in this space positively triggers a relaxation response in your body.

Safety is a primary concern for anyone, but it holds particular significance if you've experienced trauma. It's important to assess your living environment for aspects that make you feel unsafe or uneasy.

This might mean ensuring locks are sturdy and functional, using window coverings to increase privacy, or rearranging furniture to decrease feelings of vulnerability where you rest.

The addition of security cameras or motion sensors may also provide an extra layer of comfort by allowing you to monitor your surroundings.

Personalizing your space is about making your home a reflection of who you are and what brings you joy and comfort. Here are some ideas:

- Fill your space with colors that soothe or energize you, depending on your needs.
- Hang art that makes you feel happy or inspired.
- Use textiles like blankets and pillows that are comfortable and pleasing to the touch.
- Display photographs of happy memories or loved ones to create a positive atmosphere.

✓ **Each personal touch reinforces your sense of identity, allowing you to feel truly at home in your space.**

By taking steps to create a safe and healing home environment, you craft a space that supports your daily efforts in managing PTSD.

A home that aligns with your healing goals not only provides a practical environment conducive to recovery but also serves as a constant, gentle reminder of your progress and resilience.

In transforming your living space, you reaffirm your commitment to recovery and self-care, fostering a sanctuary where healing isn't just possible—it's nurtured.

Boundaries and Relationships: Navigating Social Dynamics

In a daily practice where personal growth and healing are paramount, establishing and maintaining healthy boundaries is imperative. Boundaries are not just lines drawn to keep people out.

Boundaries are personal parameters where you find freedom and safety to explore your needs and express your true self.

For those of us who have served in the military, particularly in environments where personal space and autonomy were often compromised, learning to set and respect our boundaries can be challenging and liberating.

Understanding the importance of boundaries is the first step. Personal boundaries protect your energy, minimize emotional drains, and provide a sense of individuality and respect.

When struggling with past trauma, our emotional and psychological resources are already severely taxed.

- ✓ **Establishing solid and clear boundaries is essential to manage interactions and conserve our energies for the healing process.**

Boundaries may range from deciding who you spend time with and how much time you spend with them, to what topics you are comfortable discussing, and how you allow others to treat you.

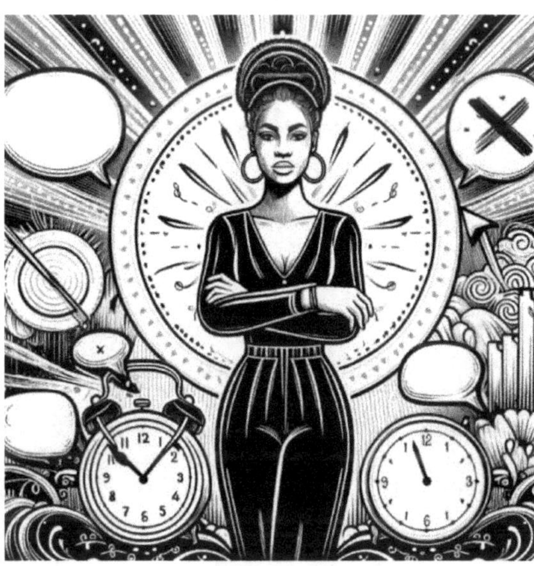

Identifying your personal boundaries is an introspective process that varies widely from person to person. Start by reflecting on past interactions that left you feeling uncomfortable, drained, or disrespected. These feelings are indicators that your boundaries were crossed.

Think about what would have needed to be different in those interactions to avoid these feelings. This reflection helps clarify where you need to set limits.

For instance, you might realize you need to limit your exposure to someone who consistently dismisses your feelings, or you may decide not to discuss certain topics, like your service or specific aspects of your PTSD, with people who aren't in your trusted circle. Effectively communicating these boundaries cannot be overstated.

- ✓ **Learning to express your needs clearly and without apology is essential to your recovery.**

Example: If someone brings up a topic that triggers you, give a clear and straightforward response. You might say, "I find it distressing to talk about that experience. Let’s discuss something else."

Assertive communication respects your feelings and those of others—it's not about being aggressive or passive. It's about being honest and direct about your needs.

Navigating difficult relationships is particularly challenging. These might be relationships that existed before your diagnosis or new ones that have become strained due to changes in your behavior as you navigate your healing process.

When a relationship consistently leaves you feeling worse off, and your boundaries are not respected despite clear communication, it may be necessary to distance yourself from that relationship. This act of distancing might be temporary or permanent, depending on the situation.

- ✓ **Distancing yourself is not a failure—it's a form of self-care.**

Building and maintaining supportive connections is equally important. These are relationships with individuals who understand and respect your boundaries, offer support and empathy, and contribute positively to your healing journey.

Cultivating such relationships might involve joining support groups for PTSD, where you connect with others who have similar experiences and understand the challenges you face. It may also mean strengthening bonds with family or friends who support you. In these relationships, mutual respect and understanding provides a foundation for emotional support and connection, which is indispensable in recovery.

Wrapping it Up

Navigating social dynamics with complex PTSD involves a delicate balance of protecting your well-being with boundaries and fostering supportive, understanding relationships.

By learning to set appropriate boundaries and communicate them effectively, you empower yourself to manage interactions proactively. This empowerment helps you build a supportive network that respects your needs and aids in your recovery, making each new day a step toward reclaiming your life and well-being.

As we conclude this exploration of creating a supportive lifestyle, let's take a moment to recap. We've examined strategies that fortify your daily life, from structuring your day for success, ensuring nutritional well-being, staying hydrated, optimizing sleep, creating a safe and healing home environment, and managing boundaries and relationships.

Each aspect weaves into the next, creating practices that support and sustain your journey toward healing.

Moving Forward

Looking ahead, the next chapter will explore mindfulness and self-compassion—elements offering deeper insights into managing PTSD symptoms and fostering enduring resilience.

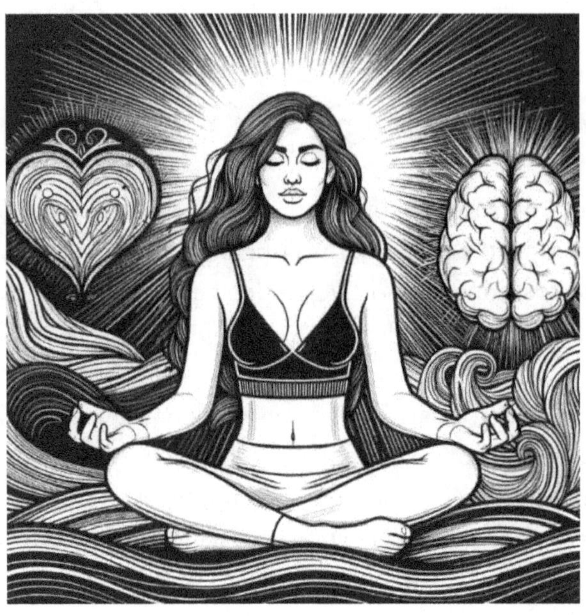

Step 8: Engage Your Mind

Practicing Mindfulness & Self Compassion

In the quiet moments of the morning, before the world stirs into its usual pace and chaos, imagine finding a peaceful clarity that centers your thoughts, soothes your nerves, and prepares you to face the day with a grounded sense of self. This practice isn't just a luxury. It's a fundamental tool.

Mindfulness, the art of present-moment awareness and acceptance, is a beacon of light in the often-tumultuous journey of healing from trauma. It teaches us to anchor ourselves in the now and offers respite from the relentless waves of memories and future anxieties.

Mindful Practices for the Present

Mindfulness is more than just a buzzword. It's a therapeutic practice that has been scientifically proven to reduce stress, anxiety, and depression—all common companions of PTSD.

At its core, mindfulness involves focusing on the present moment while calmly acknowledging and accepting your feelings, thoughts, and bodily sensations.

This seemingly simple act may be revolutionary for someone with PTSD.

- ✓ **When mindful, you observe life as it unfolds without judging or needing to change anything.**

Mindfulness is remarkably liberating. This is especially if you've spent years in hyper-vigilance, bracing for danger, reliving past traumas, or catastrophizing the future.

Mindfulness gradually teaches your brain to exit the pathways of fight, flight or freeze and enter a state of balance and reflection.

This shift is pivotal because it allows you to process your experiences in a way that leads to enhanced healing.

Simple Mindfulness Exercises

Incorporating mindfulness into your daily routine doesn't have to be daunting. Start small. Experiment with exercises that easily fit into your day-to-day activities.

Mindful eating, for example, is a practice that involves paying full attention to the experience of eating and drinking, both inside and outside the body. Notice the colors, smells, textures, and flavors of your food. Chew slowly and be aware of your body's signals of hunger and satisfaction. This practice turns a routine meal into a moment of deep presence and enjoyment.

Another accessible practice is mindful walking, which is especially beneficial if you find stillness challenging. It involves walking slowly and steadily, focusing entirely on the movement of your body and your breath.

Feel your feet touch the ground, listen to the rhythm of your breath, and notice the sensation of air on your skin. Whether walking in a busy city or a quiet hallway, the goal is to be completely in the moment.

These practices anchor you firmly in the present, providing a break from intrusive thoughts and allowing you to reconnect with your environment and body.

Mindfulness in Daily Activities

The beauty of mindfulness is that it can be integrated into virtually any activity, turning ordinary tasks into opportunities for stress relief and self-discovery.

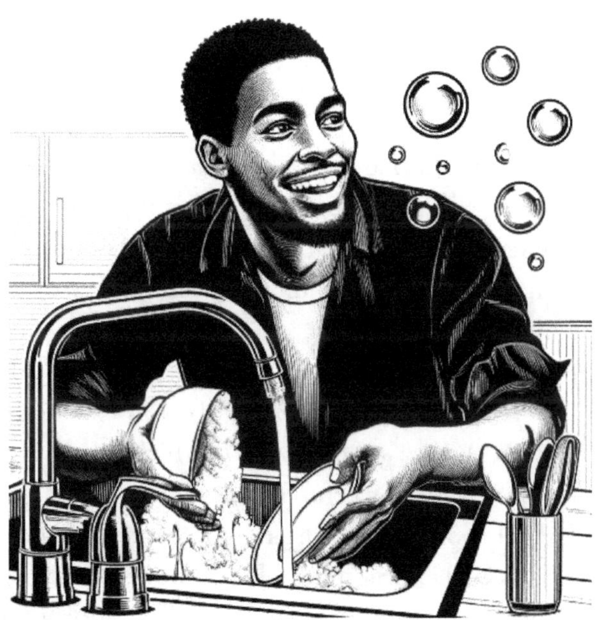

Whether you're washing dishes, taking a shower, or driving, you can practice mindfulness.

Integrating mindfulness into your daily activities transforms mundane routines into rituals of peace and presence. This integration helps build resilience, making it easier to manage PTSD symptoms as they arise.

Over time, these moments of mindfulness lead to sizable changes in how you relate to yourself and the world around you, fostering a sense of peace and stability that will be incredibly healing.

Resources for Further Practice

Numerous resources are available if you're interested in deepening your mindfulness practice. Below are just a few ideas.

Check these out:

- ❖ Check out mobile apps like *Headspace* and *Calm*, offering guided meditations and mindfulness exercises that cater to a range of needs, from anxiety management to sleep improvement.
- ❖ Books are great, too. You might enjoy these titles: *Wherever You Go, There You Are* by Jon Kabat-Zinn and *The Miracle of Mindfulness by* Thich Nhat Hanh. Both provide powerful insights and practical guidance on incorporating mindfulness into everyday life. Additionally, local mindfulness courses or workshops provide structured learning and the support of a community, which can be incredibly beneficial.

- ❖ Don't forget about Audiobooks! I love audiobooks because listening allows my restless body to keep moving. I can knock out the dirty dishes, walk, or stretch, all while learning something new. You'll find the above titles and so many more available on *Audible.*

Exploring these resources will help you tailor your mindfulness practice to meet your specific needs, enhancing your journey toward healing from PTSD.

Each step in this practice is a step toward reclaiming your life from the shadows of trauma, illuminating a path marked by peace, presence, and renewed self-connection.

Self-Compassion: Treating Yourself with Kindness

In the solitude of your own experiences, amid the echoes of a past that often seems louder than the present, self-compassion emerges as a practice and as a sanctuary.

Self-compassion is a place where you can lay down the weights of self-judgment and harshness and, instead, wrap yourself in the softness of your own kindness.

We are often so kind and compassionate to others but hard on ourselves. Why?

It makes no sense at all to leave yourself out of the equation. Now is the time to extend that same grace to yourself!

Self-compassion teaches us to treat ourselves with the same kindness, concern, and support we would offer a good friend.

- ✓ **Rebounding from complex PTSD isn't about reaching the destination of being "healed."**

There is no final finish line. Instead, recovering is an ongoing practice. It is about moving forward while nurturing yourself gently along the path.

Navigating through PTSD, especially stemming from military experiences, might often involve dealing with a harsh inner critic.

This critic keeps you trapped in a cycle of self-judgment. This not only hampers your healing but also extends your suffering.

Self-compassion shifts this narrative. It allows you to recognize that suffering and imperfection are part of the shared human experience.

- ✓ **You are not alone in your struggles, nor are you to blame for your pain.**

Embracing this perspective considerably lessens the isolation that PTSD often engenders, bridging a connection to a common humanity, a thread that binds us all in our imperfections and struggles.

Practicing self-compassion starts with simple yet sincere actions.

Write a Letter to Yourself!

Writing letters or notes to yourself helps externalize your feelings and cultivate a compassionate voice. Over time, this voice becomes a natural response to your own suffering.

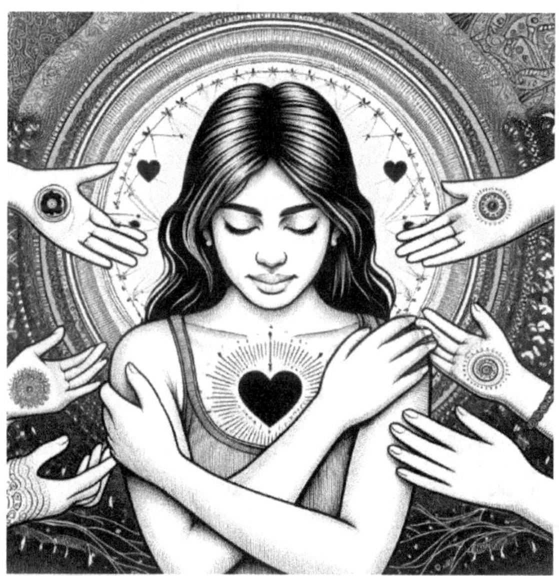

Give it a try:

- Imagine writing to a friend who is suffering.
- What words of comfort would you offer?
- How would you uplift them?
- Now, write these words to yourself.
- Address the letter to yourself, discussing your challenges.
- Acknowledge your pain.
- Offer words of support and encouragement.
- Keep this letter as a reminder and reread it often.

Another application of self-compassion is *Self-soothing*. Self-soothing skills are especially helpful in moments when your symptoms flare.

This might involve physical gestures of comfort, like placing your hands over your heart or wrapping your arms around yourself in a gentle hug.

Remember the *Butterfly Hug* we practiced earlier? The Butterfly Hug is not only a grounding tool but also an excellent method of self-soothing.

Your own gentle touch naturally elicits a soothing response from your body, releasing oxytocin and reducing cortisol levels, which helps alleviate stress and anxiety.

How can you pair touch with compassionate self-coaching? Start by putting a hand to your heart and saying, "It's okay to feel scared. I am here for you."

- ✓ **Combining gentle speech and touch reinforces that you deserve your own kindness and care.**

More than likely, this is the same kind of love and compassion you would gladly offer to others. So, give it to yourself!

Integrating Self-Compassion into Daily Life

To infuse self-compassion more deeply into your daily life, begin by setting intentions each morning.

Here are some tips to get you started:

- As you wake, spend a few moments in bed to set intentions.
- Decide to treat yourself with kindness throughout the day.
- Affirm: "Today, I will treat myself with kindness and patience."
- Now, get out of bed, wash your face, stretch, and be nice to yourself!

Setting such an intention serves as a gentle reminder throughout the day, helping to realign your actions and thoughts to a more compassionate approach.

Regularly check in with yourself. Several times throughout the day, especially during moments of stress or after a flashback, pause and ask yourself, "What do I need right now?" This question will guide you to understand and honor your needs, whether taking a break, seeking comfort in a loved one, relaxing with a cup of tea, or simply taking a few deep breaths.

Listening to and meeting your needs is a fundamental aspect of practicing self-compassion.

Celebrate your small victories. PTSD recovery is marked by countless small steps. Each time you manage a symptom better, each moment you choose self-compassion over self-judgment is a victory.

Celebrate yourself! Acknowledge your efforts and progress, no matter how small they may seem. This not only bolsters your self-esteem but also reinforces the practice of self-compassion as a valuable and effective tool in your healing arsenal.

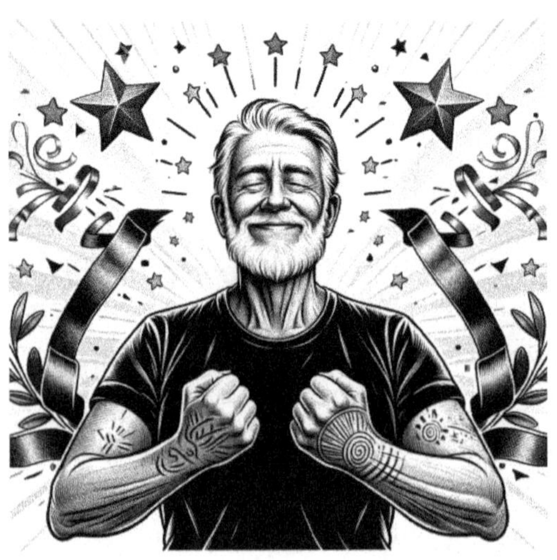

The benefits of cultivating self-compassion are numerous. Research consistently shows that self-compassion increases overall well-being, reduces symptoms of anxiety and depression, and enhances resilience.

By treating yourself with kindness, you alleviate your current suffering and build a foundation of emotional resilience that supports you throughout your life.

Resilience allows you to face challenges with a greater sense of self-assurance and composure. Become your very own ally. Equip yourself with an expanded capacity for compassion and understanding.

As you continue to integrate self-compassion into your life, remember that each act of kindness toward yourself is a remarkable step towards healing.

With each step, you move away from the pain of the past while moving toward a future where you live with greater peace, fulfillment, and self-acceptance.

Meditation Techniques for Calming the Mind

Meditation, often perceived as a practice reserved for monks or the spiritually enlightened, is actually an extremely effective tool for anyone, including those of us handling past trauma.

Meditation is not mysterious. Instead, it is about finding a quiet space within us—a refuge where the tumult of past experiences is met with a gentle, observing calm.

There are several types of meditation that can be beneficial for managing PTSD, each offering a unique approach to fostering peace and mental clarity.

Focused Attention Meditation, for instance, is a foundational practice where you focus your attention on a single point. This focus point could be your breath, a specific word or phrase (a mantra), or even a candle flame.

The goal here is not to clear the mind but to steady it, gently returning your focus to your chosen object whenever you notice it wandering.

This practice teaches you to anchor your mind in the present, reducing the power of intrusive memories or anxious thoughts about the future.

Another healing form of meditation is loving-kindness, or *Metta Meditation*, which focuses on cultivating feelings of goodwill, kindness, and warmth towards yourself and others. Start with yourself and then gradually extend that kindness to friends, family, acquaintances, and even those you may have conflicts with.

This extension especially alters your emotional response patterns because it directly counters feelings of isolation, anger, or resentment—emotions that often accompany and prolong trauma responses.

Body Scan Meditation is another effective technique, especially for those of us experiencing physical symptoms like tension, restlessness, or generalized aches and pains. In this practice, you pay attention to different parts of your body, observing without judgment.

You can start with your feet. Spend some time with your toes. Work your way up to your knees. Ask your hips how they feel today...

- ✓ **Intentionally connecting with each part of your beautiful body in a loving and nurturing way promotes relaxation and a heightened sense of bodily awareness and acceptance.**

For beginners, the world of meditation might feel as daunting as it is vast, but guided meditation can be a helpful way to start.

Guided meditation is typically led by an experienced practitioner. Sessions may be accessed through various platforms—apps, websites, and local classes.

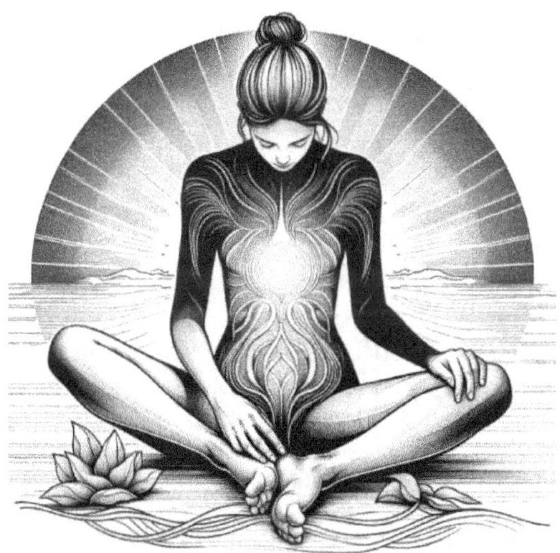

Guided meditations provide a voice to lead you through the process, offering instructions and reminders to bring your focus back when your mind wanders.

These guided meditations often include imagery, sounds, or mantras to help keep your mind engaged.

Start with a short session. Try five minutes a day.

Just five short minutes makes a sizable difference in your ability to handle stress and gradually build your confidence in your meditation practice.

Incorporating meditation into your daily life need not be a monumental task. It may be as simple as dedicating a few minutes each morning or evening to practice.

Over time, you might find that your meditation moments of calm are a cherished part of your day and something you look forward to for peace and balance.

You can also integrate micro-meditative moments throughout your day—taking a few deep breaths before starting your car. Pause for a moment of quiet before eating.

Practice a few minutes of focused attention before bedtime. It really can be that simple!

Anyone new to meditation would be wise to address common challenges and misconceptions about meditation.

A frequent hurdle is the belief that "good" meditation means having a completely empty mind. This is a myth.

- ✓ **Meditation is not about achieving emptiness. Instead, meditation is about developing awareness, presence, and compassion.**

Remember: It's normal for your mind to wander—that's just what minds do!

I call this phenomenon, *Monkey-Mind.* And trust me when I tell you, I have a very busy little monkey inhabiting my mind.

The goal here, again, is to focus on the process. Don't get frustrated. Be kind to your inner monkey!

Steps to tame the monkey:

1. Notice that your mind has wandered.
2. Just notice.
3. Do not judge.
4. Next, try gently coaxing your monkey back on-task.
5. You might say, "Oh, there you are, little monkey. That's okay. Now, let's come back over here."
6. Continue like nothing happened because nothing did.

Another challenge is the frustration that sometimes comes when results aren't immediate. Meditation is a skill that requires practice, and its benefits, while remarkable, often build gradually over time.

- ✓ **Consistency is key.**

The more regularly you practice, the more natural it will feel and the greater impact it will have on your overall well-being.

By embracing meditation, you equip yourself with a powerful tool to calm your mind, ground your thoughts, and enhance your capacity to live more fully in the present.

These moments of peace add up, contributing substantially to your healing process and offering a quiet yet intense strength to face the challenges of complex PTSD.

The Role of Gratitude in Recovery

On your road to recovery from complex PTSD, where some days feel overshadowed by memories and ongoing struggles, embracing gratitude may seem paradoxical, if not entirely out of reach.

It is in these challenging times that the practice of gratitude will shine its light most brightly, offering not just a momentary lift but a pivotal shift in how life is perceived.

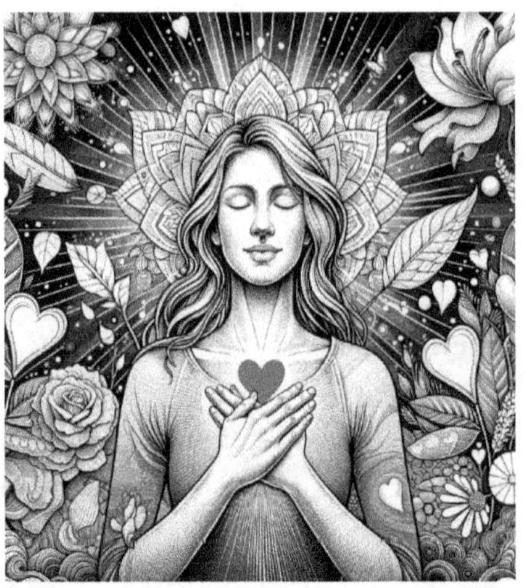

Gratitude is the recognition and appreciation of the positive aspects of life, which dramatically alters the mental landscape of someone who has experienced trauma.

Practicing gratitude is not about denying the pain or difficulties you face; rather, it's about broadening your focus to include the good alongside the challenges, which fosters resilience and a more balanced perspective on life.

The practice of gratitude has been shown to directly counteract the negativity bias—the brain's tendency to focus more readily on negative experiences than positive ones.

This bias is particularly pronounced in those of us dealing with C-PTSD, where the mind is often hypervigilant and skewed towards potential threats or painful memories.

By consciously focusing on the positive aspects of your day, gratitude helps recalibrate this bias, making the good more salient and less overshadowed by the negative.

This shift toward gratitude by no means erases the bad. Instead, it puts it into a broader context that includes joy, beauty, and connection.

One simple yet effective way to cultivate gratitude is through maintaining a gratitude journal.

Here's how to start:

1. Write down three things you are grateful for each day.
2. Focus on small things: Warm coffee in your cup, a smile, a clean kitchen...
3. Keep it simple.
4. Consistency is key!

Over time, your journaling practice helps you notice more positive moments as they occur, gradually building a habit of focusing on the positive.

Gratitude habits are powerful tools in changing how you experience the world, making it less threatening and more enriched with potential for joy and discovery.

Sharing gratitude with others also amplifies its effects. Expressing thanks to someone who has helped you or acknowledging the good you see in another not only uplifts the other person but also reinforces your own feelings of gratitude.

Spreading gratitude around will help strengthen relationships. It's like a good fertilizer for growing and strengthening your social connections and systems of support.

Expressing gratitude also shifts interactions with others from potentially conflict-focused or withdrawal-driven to more connection-oriented and positive. Try it out!

The practice of gratitude in the context of trauma recovery does come with its challenges. On difficult days, finding aspects to be grateful for may feel forced or inauthentic.

It's important to acknowledge that gratitude doesn't require denying pain or difficulty. Instead, it's about allowing yourself to recognize that alongside the bad, there are also elements of good.

This mental shift in focus is a gentle yet powerful form of self-validation, acknowledging your resilience and the complexity of your experiences.

The long-term benefits of regular gratitude practice are well-documented. Studies have shown that people who practice gratitude report fewer symptoms of illness, better sleep, more optimism, and greater happiness.

Gratitude-oriented people tend to be more resilient in the face of stress and recover more quickly from traumatic events.

As you integrate gratitude into your daily routine, you might find it becoming a natural part of your perspective, a lens that not only brightens your days but also deepens your appreciation for the nuances of your journey.

Shifting to a gratitude-focused lens offers a beacon of positivity, guiding you towards a life with the beauty and richness that define your existence.

Building Resilience through Positive Affirmations

In the quiet moments of self-reflection, it becomes apparent that the words we tell ourselves cast long shadows over our thoughts and actions.

Consider for a moment the power of language, how it shapes our reality and influences our emotional landscape.

For those of us rebounding from complex PTSD, transforming the internal dialogue is a pivotal step in reclaiming your mental space from the grips of trauma.

Positive affirmations are simple yet potent declarations about our unique selves and our amazing capabilities.

These tools are designed to challenge and rewire the negative thought patterns often entrenched by our past traumas.

The Power of Positive Affirmations

Positive affirmations are based on the principle of *neuroplasticity*—the brain's ability to reorganize itself by forming new neural connections throughout life.

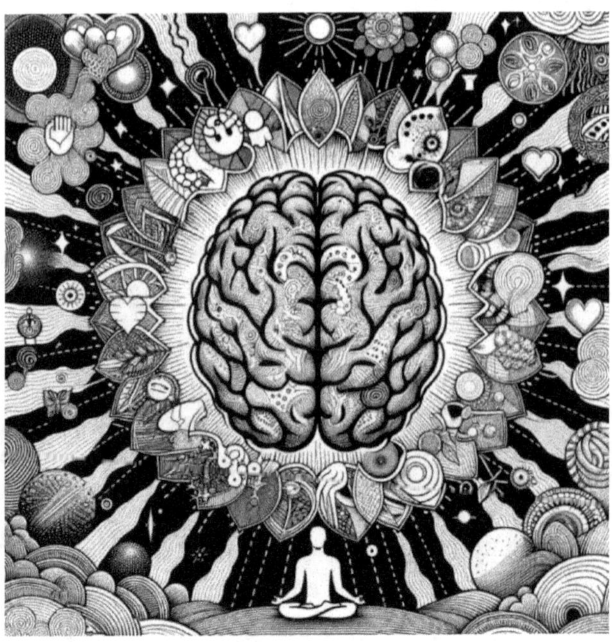

The good news behind neuroplasticity is that habitual thinking patterns can be changed, and positive affirmations are a method to facilitate this change.

Each affirmation is a conscious, positive statement that directs focus towards a desired goal or attitude, counteracting the often-automatic negative thoughts that may dominate your mind.

- ✓ **Affirmative phrases are more than just wishful thinking. These phrases are disciplined practices.**

Envisioning a different perspective cultivates a mindset that will endure the challenges posed by PTSD.

Start with simple affirmative phrases. Give it a try!

- ❖ I can move beyond my past experiences.
- ❖ I deserve love, peace, and joy.
- ❖ I am bigger than my trauma.
- ❖ I am taking charge of my recovery.
- ❖ I am brave and capable of healing.
- ❖ I am improving my health and totally kicking ass.
- ❖ I have the power to tame my triggers.
- ❖ I can outshine my anxiety.
- ❖ I am worthy of living my best life!

Affirmations are not just words—they are declarations of your intention and commitment to heal.

Your affirmative phrases remind you of your strength, ability, and worthiness.

Regularly affirm your value and capabilities. Encourage a sense of self-efficacy and resilience.

After all, you have all the essential qualities required to navigate the complexities of recovery. So, dust them off and let them shine.

Creating Personal Affirmations

While I offered a few simple examples above, try creating your own.

Affirmations unique to your own voice will resonate more deeply.

1. Start by identifying areas in your life where you feel vulnerable or challenged—perhaps it's self-esteem, trust, or optimism.

2. Reflect on these areas and write statements that directly address and transform these feelings into something positive. For example, if you struggle with self-worth, an affirmation could be, "I am worthy of love and respect."

3. Craft your affirmations in the present tense, as if they are already true. This helps you begin to accept them as reality.

4. Keep affirmations clear and simple.

5. Ensure your words evoke a positive emotional response when you say them. This emotional connection reinforces their impact and makes the practice more rewarding.

6. Integrate your affirmations into your daily routine. This will enhance the overall effectiveness of your words.

7. Start in the morning. Say an affirmation before getting out of bed.

8. Try looking into a mirror while getting yourself ready. Give yourself a big smile and say something positive.

9. Put an affirmation-loaded sticky note on your coffee pot. Or better yet, get your affirmation printed on a mug.

10. Stick brightly colored, affirmative Post-it notes throughout your living space.

11. Create an affirmation background on your phone and laptop.

While these steps seem quite simple and somewhat corny, they serve as helpful reminders to engage in your affirmation practice throughout the day, especially when negative thoughts invade your space.

Overcoming Skepticism

It's natural to be skeptical about the effectiveness of positive affirmations, particularly if you're accustomed to a critical or pessimistic mindset.

This skepticism, while valid, can be a barrier to experiencing the benefits of this practice.

- ✓ **Move past skepticism by considering the research. Better yet, conduct your own research!**

If you conduct your own research, you will discover that affirmations are indeed supportive of our efforts to improve our mental health.

You'll find no shortage of scholarly, peer-reviewed articles on the topic.

You'll uncover study after study indicating noteworthy correlations between positive self-statements, decreased stress, and increased feelings of self-worth.

Why Not Conduct Your Own Experiment?

1. Approach affirmations with an open mind, a bit of humor, and a spirit of investigation.

2. Try them consistently for a few weeks.

3. Check in with yourself daily to monitor any shifts in your mood or thought patterns.

As you integrate positive affirmations into your life, remember that each repetition is an act of building, of laying down new pathways in your brain that affirm your strength, resilience, and worth.

This practice doesn't just help reshape your internal dialogue; it opens new possibilities for how you live and engage with the world.

- ✓ **Life-affirming statements build a foundation of positive beliefs to support your journey of recovery and growth.**

Wrapping it Up

In this chapter, we've explored how engaging mindfulness and adding techniques like meditation channels, expressions of gratitude, and positive affirmations into your daily routine will greatly impact your recovery journey.

Practicing meditation, expressing gratitude, and reciting affirmation statements are all simple, cost-free ways to reshape negative thought patterns and foster resilience.

As we close this discussion, remember that each positive statement, each kind word of compassion, and every expression of gratitude is a step forward in rediscovering the strength and value you hold within.

Embrace this section as part of a broader spectrum of strategies designed to support your healing.

Each step contributes to a holistic approach that honors your passage through trauma and supports your growth.

Moving Forward

Looking ahead, the next chapter will explore deeper into strategies for maintaining momentum in your healing journey.

These strategies work to ensure that the practices and insights you've gained so far will continue to empower you toward a fuller, more vibrant life.

- ✓ **Setbacks are a normal part of our journey. Learning to navigate these moments is imperative.**

Continuity checks are not just about overcoming past pain but about building a future filled with hope and fulfillment.

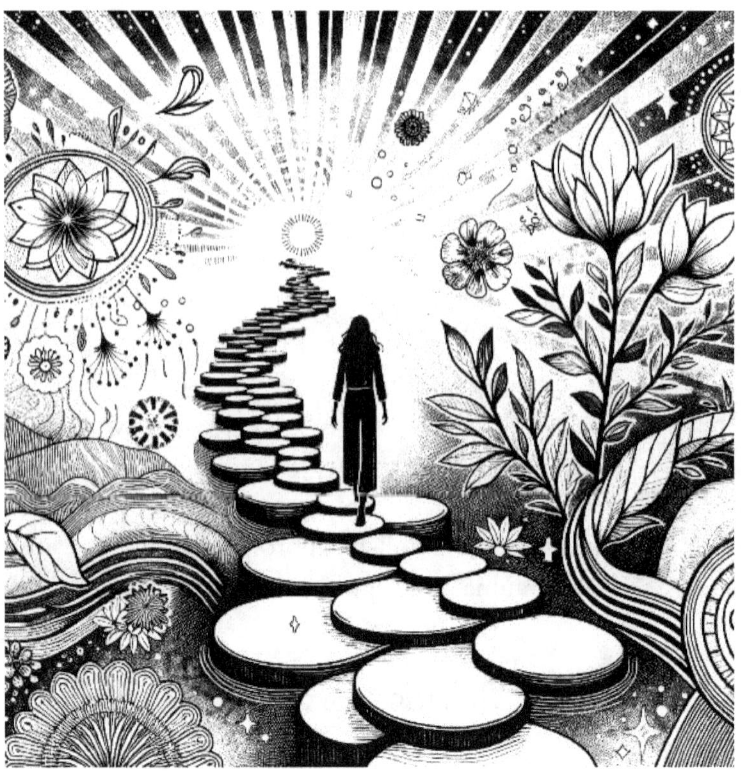

Step 9: Navigate Setbacks & Challenges

Imagine you're walking through a maze. The path ahead twists and turns, making each corner a new challenge. Perhaps you'll face a roadblock. That's okay. Turn yourself around and try another route. Eventually, you'll find the path of discovery.

In this metaphorical maze we call *life*, you'll sometimes find yourself at a standstill, a quiet clearing where the path seems to level out, and the scenery becomes monotonously familiar.

This is much like encountering a healing plateau in your journey with complex PTSD—a phase where, despite your efforts, the progress seems to stall, leaving you questioning your strategies or even the possibility of further recovery.

Rest assured. In these quiet clearings, these plateaus, you'll find the space to take a moment, reassess, gather strength, and gear up for the next leg of your odyssey.

Identifying and Overcoming Plateaus

A healing plateau sometimes feels like you're running into an invisible barrier that no amount of effort will penetrate.

You might recall the initial stages of your recovery, moments filled with major breakthroughs, where each day seemed to bring a new revelation or improvement. But now, progress feels elusive, and the transformative pace that once energized you feels like a distant memory.

- ✓ **Please understand that these plateaus are a natural part of the healing process.**

Plateaus do not signify a regression or failure but rather a pause, an essential respite for your mind and body to absorb the changes you have undergone.

In the context of complex PTSD, especially for veterans who have lived through meticulously structured and often high-stakes environments, the lack of visible progress might be particularly disheartening.

Although plateaus are frustrating, plateaus are perfectly normal. Just as the body sometimes needs to rest after a long march to rebuild strength, so does the psyche need its moments of stillness to integrate new strategies and lessons learned.

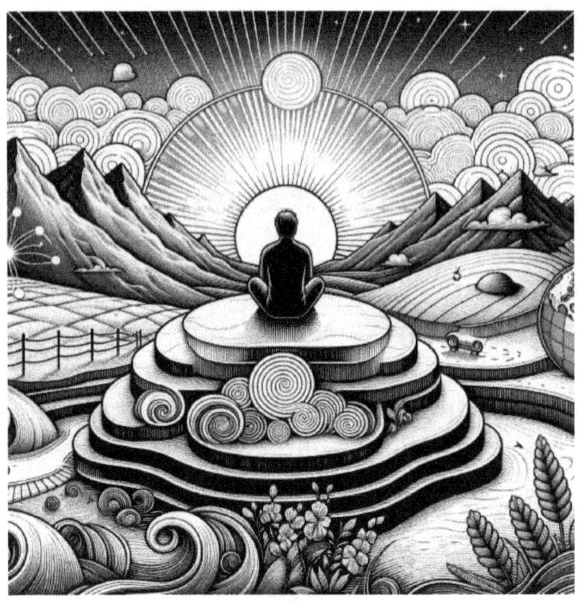

Recognizing Signs of a Plateau

Identifying a plateau involves carefully reflecting on your recent state of mind and emotions. You might feel stuck or wonder if the strategies that previously propelled you forward are still effective.

Check in with yourself. Look for signs indicating a pervasive sense of stagnation, diminished motivation, or a feeling that you're merely *going through the motions* without experiencing the emotional or psychological growth you expect.

You might also notice decreased enthusiasm towards your therapy sessions or self-help activities. Therapeutic activities that used to spark a sense of hope or curiosity now seem routine or uninspiring.

Strategies to Overcome Plateaus

Start by reviewing your current treatment strategies with your therapist or support group. An open conversation about your feelings of stagnation may lead to adjustments in your therapy or an introduction of new approaches to reignite your progress.

- ✓ **Breaking through a plateau requires patience, adjustment, and sometimes a bit of creativity.**

Example: If your current regimen is heavily focused on talk therapy, integrating art therapy or mindfulness practices might provide new avenues for expression and insight.

Engaging in new hobbies or activities also stimulates mental and emotional growth, pushing you gently off the plateau.

Whether it's learning a new skill, exploring a new place, or simply altering your routine, change challenges your brain in beneficial ways and invigorates your recovery process.

These activities don't have to be grand or daunting. Even small changes will make a big difference!

Maintaining Perspective

Most importantly, maintain perspective on what a plateau represents. It's not a sign that you've reached the limits of your recovery, or that future progress is unattainable. Rather, it's a natural and expected part of the healing journey.

- ✓ **Every recovery is non-linear. It is marked by ebbs, flows, peaks, and valleys.**

Remind yourself that this plateau can be a period of consolidation, where gains are solidified, and strategies are recalibrated.

Remember, the path through a maze is not a straight line but a series of twists and turns, each leading to new vistas.

Similarly, your healing path is dynamic, and each plateau is simply a pause, a moment to catch your breath before moving forward to new challenges and triumphs.

Dealing with Relapses: A Guide to Getting Back on Track

In the landscape of recovering from complex PTSD, envisioning a relapse can be likened to a sudden storm disrupting a period of calm weather.

You might find old symptoms resurfacing or old coping mechanisms creeping back into your life despite feeling like you had them well under control.

It's important to understand that relapse in the context of PTSD recovery doesn't erase your progress or mean you must start over. Instead, it's a part of the healing process, much like those unexpected storms, reminding us that our environments and reactions are continually changing.

A relapse might manifest as a return of intense flashbacks, increased anxiety, avoidance behaviors, or perhaps a reversion to less healthy coping mechanisms like substance use or withdrawal from social contacts.

These signs can be disheartening but recognizing them early is the first step toward regaining control.

It's like noticing dark clouds gathering on the horizon and preparing yourself before the storm hits rather than being caught off-guard.

- ✓ **The cornerstone of managing challenging phases involves consistent self-care and vigilant monitoring of your mental state.**

Regular self-care routines, such as sufficient sleep, balanced nutrition, regular physical activity, and mindfulness practices, create a robust foundation for sustaining yourself during tougher times.

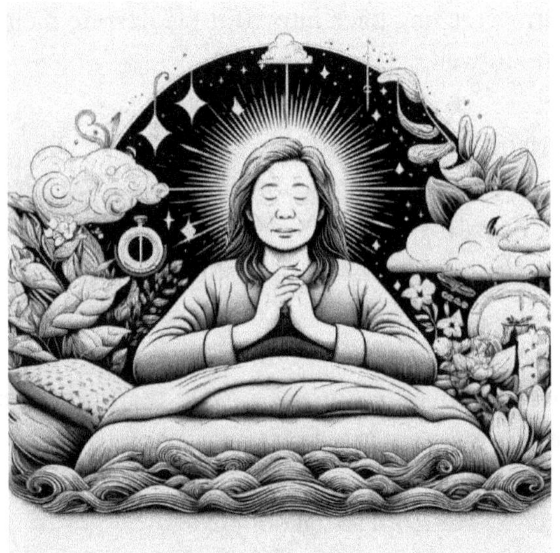

Self-monitoring involves staying dialed into your emotional and psychological states, which helps you catch and address potential triggers or stressors before they lead to a relapse.

Tools like mood trackers or journals are instrumental in this ongoing monitoring, allowing you to spot patterns or changes in your emotional landscape that might signify an approaching relapse.

When a relapse occurs, the immediate steps you take will influence the duration and intensity of this phase.

First and foremost, reach out for support. Contacting your therapist, a trusted friend, or a support group not only provides you with immediate emotional support but also helps in strategizing a response to manage and overcome the relapse.

These supports act as your anchor, helping stabilize your emotions and guiding you through turbulent times.

- ✓ **Viewing relapses as learning opportunities will transform these challenging experiences into valuable insights.**

Each relapse reveals what triggers you, which strategies are effective, and what areas might still need attention and work.

Example: If a relapse occurs after a particularly stressful week at work, it might indicate the need for more robust stress management strategies or a reevaluation of your work environment.

By analyzing what happened before and during the relapse, you can adjust your coping strategies to better manage similar situations in the future, thus strengthening your resilience against potential relapses.

These insights and realizations are often best achieved through reflection and discussion, either with your therapist or within a support group. Such reflective practices help you understand the complex patterns of your thoughts and behaviors and how they interact with your environment to influence your well-being.

Foster a kinder, more forgiving attitude towards yourself and your recovery process. Recognize that relapses are not failures but part of the healing landscape. This will allow you to navigate future setbacks with greater ease and confidence.

Framing setbacks constructively shifts your focus from a path defined by fear of relapse to one marked by growth, learning, and continual adaptation.

Each step you take, each strategy you adopt, and each support you seek helps you craft your unique response to current and future challenges, paving the way for a resilient, responsive approach to recovery.

Handling PTSD Symptoms in Public Spaces

Navigating through the hustle and bustle of public spaces often feels like a high-stakes obstacle course, especially when you're managing symptoms of complex PTSD.

The sensory overload, the unpredictability of crowds, and the sudden loud noises can all trigger a simple outing into a challenging ordeal.

It's not just the fear of potential triggers but also the feeling of being exposed and vulnerable in a public setting that works to intensify anxiety.

Understanding these unique challenges is the first step toward developing strategies for engaging with the world more confidently and securely.

Preparing for outings requires thoughtful planning, not just about the logistics of where and when to go, but also about how to create a safety net for yourself.

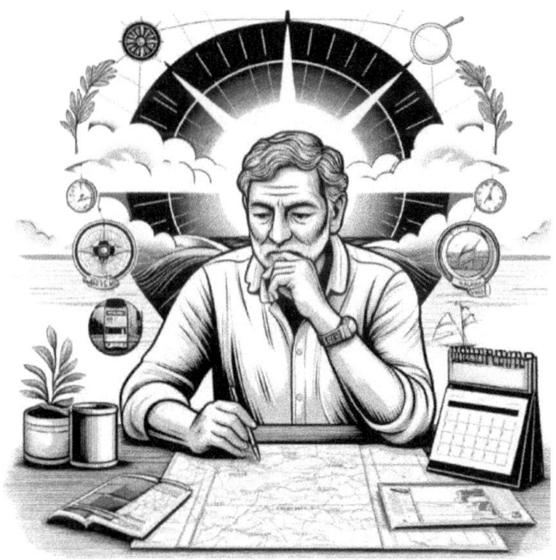

Begin by choosing times and locations that are likely to be less crowded and thus less overwhelming.

Example: Early morning hours or weekdays might be ideal for running errands or enjoying a park.

Familiarize yourself with the layout of places you plan to visit—knowing the locations of exits, restrooms, and quiet areas helps provide a sense of control and ease some of the anxiety.

Carrying a *grounding kit* is also incredibly helpful. My kit varies depending on where I plan to visit. However, there are some comfort items I always ensure are in my bag: dark sunglasses, ear plugs, and my tangerine (for smell).

Your kit will be designed by you and respond to your comforts. You might include soothing items such as headphones to listen to calming music or audiobooks, sunglasses to reduce the harshness of bright lights, or a small object, like a smooth stone or a stress ball, that you can touch to center yourself during moments of distress.

Additionally, having a plan in place in case you start feeling overwhelmed will make a measurable difference. This might involve a breathing routine, texting a friend, or using an app to guide you through grounding exercises.

While planning doesn't eliminate the possibility of encountering triggers, it does equip you with the strategies to handle them more effectively.

Once you find yourself in a public space, having strategies to manage symptoms as they arise can save the day. Begin by grounding yourself in your environment.

Try the 5-4-3-2-1 technique we discussed earlier—identify five things you can see, four you can touch, three you can hear, two you can smell, and one you can taste.

- ✓ **The incredibly simple 5-4-3-2-1 method helps you focus on your surroundings and away from the source of anxiety.**

If you feel a panic attack brewing or if flashbacks start to surface, focus on controlled breathing. Inhale through your nose slowly for four seconds, hold for four seconds, and then exhale for four seconds. This pattern helps regulate your heart rate and reduce the intensity of your symptoms.

It's also helpful to have an exit strategy planned. Sometimes, a public space becomes too overwhelming despite your best efforts. It's okay to leave and try again another day. Allowing yourself this option reduces the pressure and anxiety associated with outings, making them more manageable.

Building confidence in navigating public spaces is a gradual process. Start small—perhaps by visiting a nearby park or a quiet cafe—and gradually increase your exposure as your confidence grows.

Celebrating small victories is important. Successfully spending time in a public setting, even if it's just for a short period, is a momentous achievement and should be recognized as such. Over time, these small successes will build your confidence, making larger and busier spaces feel more accessible.

Remember, managing PTSD symptoms in public doesn't mean completely conquering your anxiety. Instead, it's about learning to navigate it in ways that make your world bigger and more engaging.

Each outing and each step you take forward is a testament to your resilience and commitment to reclaiming your freedom and joy in public spaces.

Finding and Using Professional Help

Knowing when it's time to seek professional help after a setback is an essential aspect of your journey. Often, we try to push through on our own until things become unmanageable. This is especially true if we have been making gains just before the setback.

Recognizing early signs that indicate the need for professional intervention will prevent a more severe relapse. If you find your symptoms increasingly interfering with your daily life—such as persistent anxiety, disruptive sleep patterns, flashbacks, or a feeling of being constantly on edge—it might be time to seek help.

If you notice you're relying heavily on unhealthy coping mechanisms like substance abuse or withdrawal from social interactions, these are clear indicators that professional support could be beneficial.

- ✓ **Remember, reaching out for help is a sign of strength and a proactive step in taking control of your life and health.**

Integrating professional help with self-help strategies creates a more robust approach to managing PTSD.

While therapy provides tailored strategies and a professional perspective, self-help techniques such as mindfulness, regular physical activity, and maintaining a healthy routine will radically support your therapy work.

Discuss with your therapist about integrating these practices into your treatment plan. They may offer guidance on how to align these practices with your therapeutic goals, creating a cohesive strategy that supports your overall well-being.

Example: If you're learning stress management techniques in therapy, practicing yoga or meditation will enhance those skills. Integrating holistic strategies allows you to take a more proactive role and flex self-agency in your recovery.

Locating mental health services might initially seem like deciphering a complex map with multiple routes and destinations. It's understandable to feel overwhelmed, especially when seeking someone to trust with your most vulnerable thoughts and experiences.

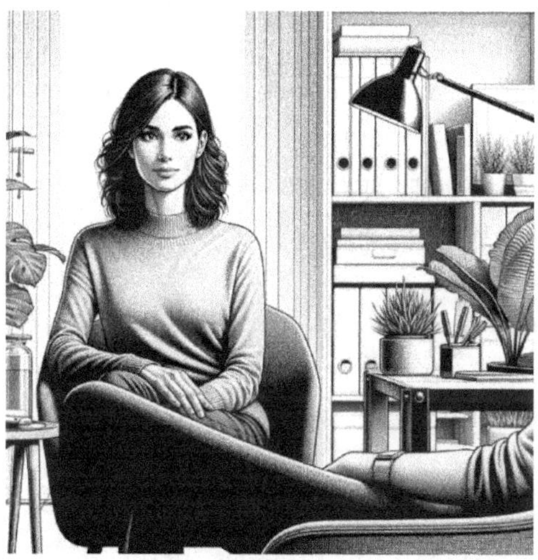

The first step in this process is identifying qualified mental health professionals who are not only skilled but also a good match for your specific needs.

The key is to focus on finding therapists who specialize in trauma and PTSD, as they will have a deeper understanding and more tools to address the nuances of your experiences.

You might start by searching through professional directories offered by reputable organizations such as the *American Psychological Association* or local veteran affairs offices that provide lists of therapists with specialized training in dealing with trauma, PTSD, and more specifically, C-PTSD.

When choosing a therapist, there are many things to consider.

Here are a few to get you started:

1. Consider their approaches: Talk therapy, EMDR, Somatic Experiencing, Art therapy...
2. Do these approaches align with your preferences?
3. If you're a veteran, does the therapist have experience with military clients?
4. What is their experience with PTSD and C-PTSD?
5. Following an initial consultation, gauge your comfort level.
6. Don't hesitate to ask questions and express your needs.
7. **Transparency is key.**

Overcoming barriers to seeking help is often one of the most challenging aspects of this process. Stigma, particularly in military communities, may seem like a major hurdle, especially when signs of vulnerability might be misinterpreted as weakness.

Recognize and challenge these misconceptions.

- ✓ **Seeking help is a wise and courageous decision. Be wise! Be courageous!**

Financial constraints might also pose a barrier. Many therapists offer sliding scale fees based on income. If you have health insurance, you might find that your policy covers part or all mental health services.

If you're a veteran, remember to reach out to the VA or other veteran-affiliated organizations like the *Disabled American Veterans* (DAV). There are programs specifically designed and funded to support the mental health of former service members.

If previous negative experiences with therapy have made you hesitant, consider giving it another chance. Keep in mind that not all therapists are the same. It's imperative to find the right match for your needs.

Navigating mental health services effectively requires patience, perseverance, and a willingness to advocate for your needs. If you feel overwhelmed, tap into your support system for assistance.

Each step towards finding and using professional help is a stride toward a more supported and sustainable recovery.

Remember, the right therapist can provide invaluable assistance. They can help you unravel emotions and guide you through the recovery process of PTSD.

When Family and Friends Don't Understand

The path to healing from complex PTSD may feel isolated, particularly when those closest to you struggle to grasp the depth of your experience.

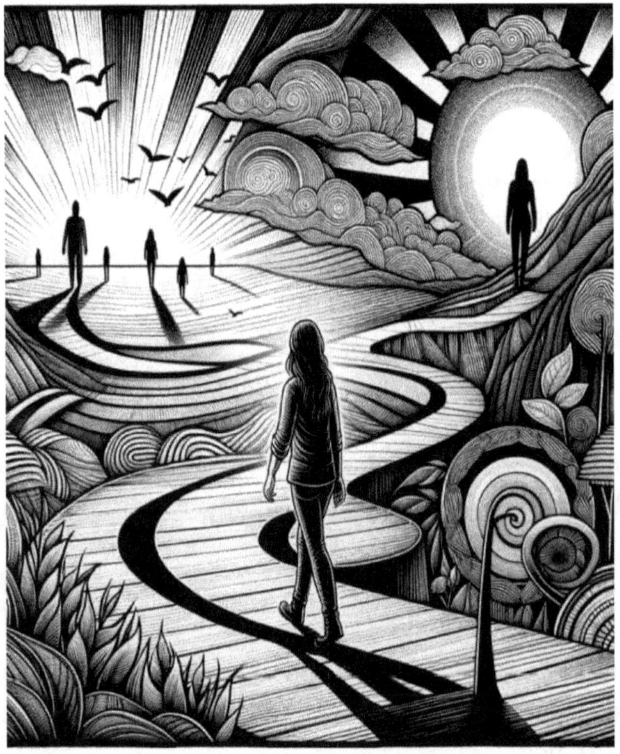

It's not uncommon for family and friends to misunderstand or even disbelieve the impacts of PTSD, especially when its manifestations aren't outwardly visible.

This gap in understanding deepens feelings of isolation and may even hinder your healing process, as the environments that should be your safest may feel subtly adversarial.

You might have tried explaining what it feels like to move through daily life with PTSD. Or maybe, you described the triggers and the exhaustive energy required to maintain a semblance of normalcy.

Regardless of your efforts to communicate with your family and friends, your explanations may be met with blank stares, dismissal, or misplaced advice. All of this only works to compound frustration and loneliness.

- ✓ **Communicating about PTSD effectively to those who may not have experienced it firsthand is difficult, to say the least.**

Here are some tips:

- Start by choosing a quiet, private time when you're unlikely to be interrupted.
- Explain PTSD or C-PTSD in very clinical terms.
- Next, try breaking the clinical jargon down into easy-to-understand concepts.
- Then, explain how these concepts relate personally to you and how you experience the world.
- Be very specific! Describe how it affects your thoughts, feelings, and behaviors.
- Explain a flashback as not simply a memory but an immersive reliving of a past trauma.
- Explain some of the things that trigger your flashbacks. Be specific: smells, sounds, scenes...
- Emphasize that flashbacks are not choices you make. Instead, they are involuntary responses your body and mind are working through.

- When explaining the type of support you need, be clear about what is helpful and what is not.
- Ask for what you need. Example: Support can be as simple as giving you space when needed.
- Set and communicate boundaries around discussing your trauma.
- Clarify what you are comfortable sharing and when.
- Explain that being pushed to discuss details can be retraumatizing.
- Encourage independent research. Recommend resources such as this and other books, audiobooks, websites, YouTube clips, and podcasts.

Wrapping it Up

Setting boundaries is an essential step in managing relationships while learning to master C-PTSD.

These boundaries might relate to your need for space during high-stress periods or controlling the conversation topics when certain subjects trigger your symptoms.

It's okay to assertively communicate your needs. Start by saying, "I find it overwhelming to talk about my experiences. I appreciate your interest. I will share more when I'm ready."

- ✓ **Boundaries aren't just about creating barriers. Boundaries are also about forging a space where healing may occur without external pressures.**

Seeking support outside your immediate social circles may also provide the understanding and validation that might be lacking at home.

Support groups, either in-person or online, connect you with others experiencing similar challenges.

These groups provide a platform to share your experiences without judgment, learn coping strategies from other survivors, and reinforce solidarity.

- ✓ **Remember: You are never alone.**

Therapists specialized in PTSD offer professional guidance and support that friends and family are unable to provide.

Professional support helps you navigate the complexities of symptoms and your recovery in a structured, supportive environment.

In these interactions with family, friends, and support systems, it's necessary to remember that misunderstanding often stems from a knowledge gap rather than a lack of care.

With patience and open communication, you can help bridge this gap.

Bridging the gap allows you to build a supportive network that understands and respects your journey toward recovery.

Moving Forward

This chapter focused on navigating the misunderstandings often encountered in personal relationships. Key takeaways include the importance of clear communication, establishing boundaries, and seeking supportive communities.

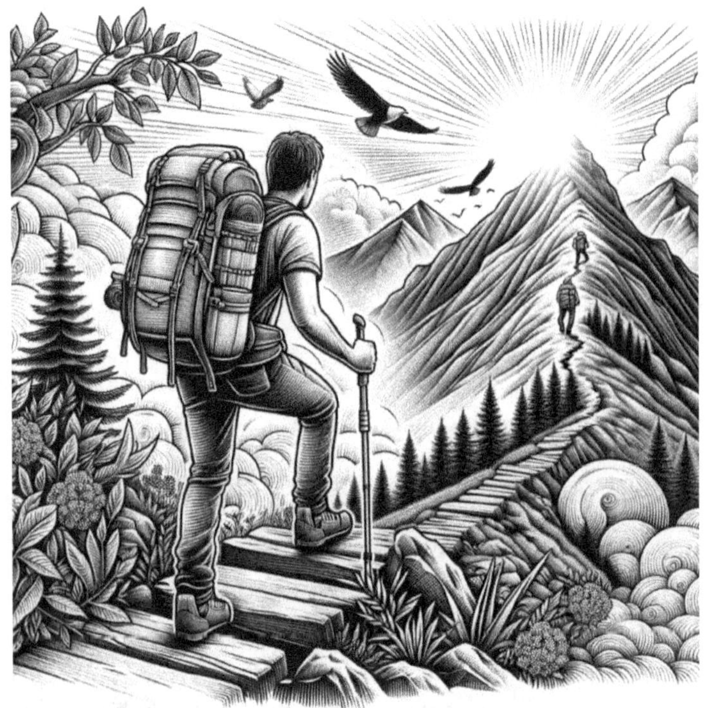

As we continue, our next steps will explore the importance of maintaining resilience when embracing future challenges. This will ensure that the strategies and insights gained are integrated into a sustainable approach to living with and, eventually, beyond PTSD and C-PTSD.

Step 10: Live Your Best Life

Imagine standing together in a beautiful valley at the edge of a vast, golden landscape. Silently, we take it all in.

Lush green forests and majestic purple mountains flank each side of our view. Ahead, a beyond-blue horizon stretches out endlessly before us.

Each step forward into that golden valley is a testament to our resilience and to our collective commitment to navigate the terrain of recovery from complex PTSD.

As we stand there with our guidebooks in hand, we realize the importance of identifying meaningful landmarks and points of progress.

We know these landmarks and progress points as our guides. These elements motivate, inspire, and keep us on track.

This is the essence of setting goals in your recovery process:

- Goals are landmarks and points of progress.
- The landmark provides direction.
- The point of progress helps measure your journey.
- Together, these elements transform a daunting path into a series of achievable steps, leading to a fuller, more powerful life.

Setting Realistic Goals for Your Recovery

Setting goals is akin to drawing a map for a journey. The process provides direction to help you focus when the path becomes difficult or your motivation wanes.

Recovery goals are tools to scaffold day-to-day and long-term recovery efforts. Goals help structure your healing process, making an often-overwhelming trek more manageable.

Each goal achieved is another building block to reconstruct your sense of self. Each building block delivers you further from the shadows of trauma.

SMART Goals for Recovery

If you have served in the military, you are probably no stranger to SMART goals. But sometimes, a refresher is required.

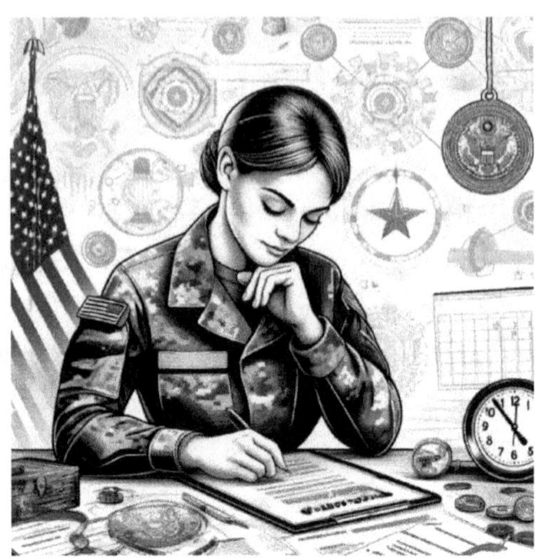

- ✓ **Important: regardless of service status, SMART goals are useful for everyone.**

Smart Criteria. Check it out:

1. Specific.
2. Measurable.
3. Achievable.
4. Relevant.
5. Time-bound.

Tried and true, SMART goals exponentially increase your chances of success.

Example 1: "I want to feel better." This goal is commendable but way too vague.

Example 2: "I want to reduce my anxiety by practicing mindfulness for 10 minutes every day and keeping a daily mood journal over the next 30 days."

The redefined goal hits all the SMART principles, making your goal clear and actionable.

Let's break down the revised goal:

1. **Specific**: Reduce Anxiety.
2. **Measurable**: Practice 10 minutes per day and create a daily entry in a mood-journal.
3. **Achievable**: Use Mindfulness and journaling as tools.
4. **Relevant**: Owning less anxiety would be wonderful!
5. **Time Bound**: 30 days.

The SMART method sets a clear expectation, provides a measurable and timely framework, helps keep you accountable, and allows you to see your progress.

Why not take a moment now and jot down a SMART goal of your own design?

Adjusting Goals as Needed

Flexibility in goal setting is required. Remember, you need to set goals to track progress and motivate, but not at the risk of abandoning self-compassion or your safety.

Understand that your day-to-day experiences will vary widely. If your goal of practicing 10 minutes of mindfulness goes in the toilet on Day 3, that's okay. Don't abandon the rest of the month. Pick right back up on Day 4 and power through.

Your goals must accommodate good days and days when your symptoms might feel insurmountable.

Example: Let's say you plan to walk 10 minutes a day. But on the 5th day, you feel so good you want to keep walking. Well, keep walking!

There's nothing wrong with being an overachiever! This is especially true when you are being so kind to yourself by moving that beautiful body of yours. **Just keep walking**!

Maintaining adaptability means setting challenging yet achievable goals and being prepared to adjust them up or down as your recovery progresses.

- ✓ **Wise goal setting is about creating a balance that encourages growth without setting you up for frustration or failure.**

Celebrating Achievements

Don't forget to celebrate every landmark and point of progress. Every step forward, no matter how small, deserves recognition.

Celebrating your achievements builds self-esteem and reinforces your commitment to recovery. Celebrations can be simple, like taking a moment to acknowledge your effort, journaling your experience, or sharing your progress with a supportive friend or therapist.

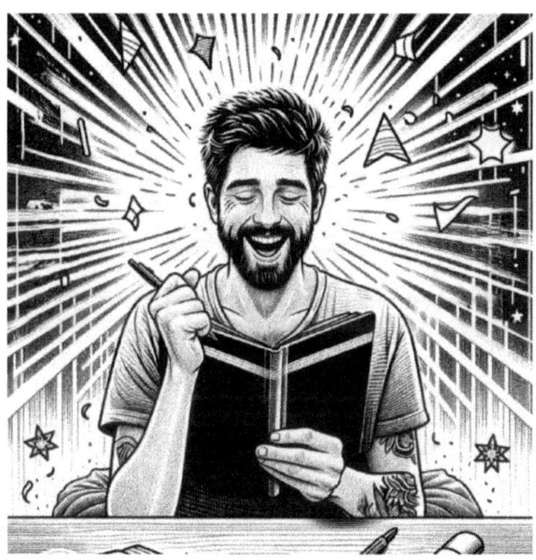

Acts of personal recognition are essential as they not only boost your morale but also remind you of your capabilities and resilience. Go ahead! Celebrate yourself!

Each success, small or great, is a milestone marking your path of recovery. Each one is a testament to your courage and determination.

As you integrate these goal-setting strategies into the fabric of your recovery, they become more than just objectives. They transform into beacons of hope—personal testaments to your ability to influence your healing and shape your future.

This brand of empowerment is fundamental not just for surviving but for thriving despite the challenges posed by complex PTSD.

As you continue to set, adjust, and achieve your goals, you gradually build a life defined not by trauma but by resilience, achievement, and fulfillment.

The Role of Hope

In the ebb and flow of living with complex PTSD, hope is not just a fleeting feeling. It is your motor, the force propelling you forward even on days shrouded in the fog of doubt and despair.

Harnessing hope involves more than mere wishful thinking. It requires nurturing a mindset that sees beyond current struggles. Hope knows healing and growth are attainable.

Hope is the belief that recovery isn't just a possibility but an expectation. It is knowing that with each step you take, you are moving toward a life defined not by trauma but by your strength and resilience.

To gather hope, begin by setting your sights on small, immediate targets. Gradually build the path to larger aspirations.

A show of hope could be as simple as deciding to make your bed each morning. This small act instills a sense of accomplishment and order at the start of your day.

- ✓ **Single acts propel you forward. These acts are steppingstones of hope, proving that change is possible.**

The power of visualization also plays a vital role in nurturing hope. Visualization allows you to see yourself not as you are right now but as you will be in the very near future.

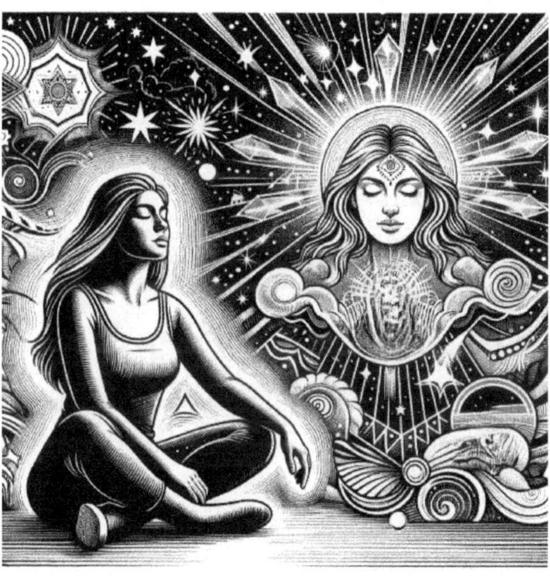

- ✓ **Spend a few moments each day envisioning your life as you wish it to be.**

Picture yourself handling a situation that currently feels overwhelming with calm and confidence. Imagine a day where peace and contentment are your prevailing emotions.

Visualization not only bolsters your spirit but also redirects your subconscious mind toward achieving these envisioned outcomes. This makes the visions more attainable.

Remember, affirmations serve as daily reminders of your potential and progress. Phrases like "I am healing a little more each day" or "I am stronger than my challenges" are powerful motivators.

Affirmations reinforce your belief in your ability to overcome the effects of PTSD. This embeds the seeds of hope in your daily thoughts and interactions.

Hope is not always a constant presence. Hope requires nurturing, especially during challenging times when despair seems more accessible than optimism. During such periods, lean into your support system. Friends, family, therapists, or support groups may provide the external affirmation necessary to reignite your internal hope.

- ✓ **Sharing your fears and frustrations openly with those who understand provides relief and brings new perspectives.**

Sometimes, just hearing someone say, "I believe in you," is all you need to lift yourself out of despair.

Remembering past achievements is also vital during times of doubt. Reflect on moments when you overcame difficulties or achieved goals, no matter how small.

These memories are proof of your ability to navigate challenges. These memories are a reservoir of strength and hope.

Hope is not just the expectation of a better tomorrow. Instead, it is the recognition of your role in creating your future. Take one small, hopeful step at a time.

Volunteer: Giving Back as a Path to Healing

In the colorful canvas of recovery, each brushstroke carries its own texture and color, contributing uniquely to the overarching design. Among these, volunteering emerges as a vibrant splash of color, enhancing both the design and the designer.

When you give your time and energy to a cause outside of yourself, your efforts benefit more than just the recipients. They benefit you!

The very act of volunteering bolsters your mental health, offering a renewed sense of purpose, deeper community connections, and an improved self-image.

- ✓ **Volunteering provides a unique opportunity to step outside of your experiences and immerse yourself by helping others.**

This shift in focus can be incredibly therapeutic. It's a chance to engage in something larger than your struggles. This helps put trauma into a broader perspective.

Moreover, the social aspect of volunteering allows you to connect with others, which will be particularly helpful if you've felt isolated by your experiences with C-PTSD.

These connections lead to increased feelings of belonging and an improved support network, which are essential elements in any recovery process.

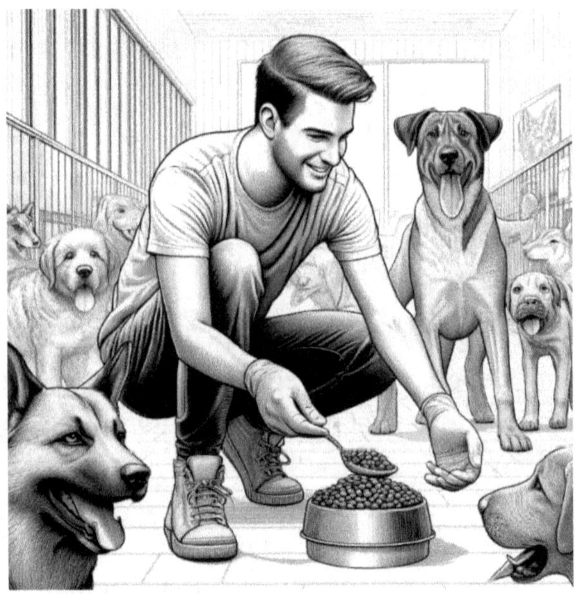

Additionally, the positive feedback and appreciation you receive as a volunteer boosts self-esteem. This reaffirms your capabilities and worth, feelings that are often overshadowed by the challenges of C-PTSD.

Finding the right volunteering opportunity is like choosing a role in a play. You want something that resonates with your interests, uses your strengths, and accommodates your current capacity. But how do you choose?

Here are some tips:

1. Consider causes you feel passionate about: wildlife, pets, environmental concerns, social services…

2. Check with local nonprofits, food banks, shelters, hospitals, and community centers. These places can offer a range of volunteering opportunities.

3. Research! Websites like VolunteerMatch.org help connect you with projects that match your interests.

4. Be honest about time commitment and what kinds of activities you feel capable of handling. Clarity will help you find a rewarding role.

5. Set healthy boundaries to ensure your volunteer work remains a positive aspect of your life.

6. Start slowly. Try not to overcommit out of enthusiasm or a desire to escape. Overcommitting leads to burnout, stress, and exacerbates symptoms.

7. Volunteering should be a fulfilling addition to your life, not a source of additional pressure.

- ✓ **The sense of community that volunteering fosters is often its most healing aspect.**

Being part of a team and working towards a common goal rebuilds the sense of connection and trust that is often strained during recovery.

The regular interaction and teamwork involved provide a social rhythm that is comforting and reassuring, a contrast to the isolation that often accompanies trauma.

Over time, these positive interactions reinforce a more hopeful outlook on life, contributing to a broader sense of belonging and community integration.

By weaving volunteering into your recovery process, you are doing more than just giving back. You are also opening a pathway to enhance your mental health by forging valuable connections and rediscovering a sense of purpose.

Remember, each act of volunteering adds a vibrant splash of color to your recovery canvas, enhancing the composition of your life and the community around you.

Speaking Out: Sharing Your Story Safely

When you choose to share your experiences of trauma and recovery, you do more than recount a personal history. You open the door to understanding and connection that deeply impacts yourself and others.

Speaking about your recovery experiences with C-PTSD serves as a powerful catalyst for change, not just in your life but in the lives of others who hear your story and see a reflection of their own struggles and hopes.

Sharing Demystifies PTSD and C-PTSD.

Sharing breaks down the walls of stigma and builds bridges of empathy and support, particularly among veterans. This is especially significant for survivors of sexual trauma where experiences, often shrouded by shame, go unspoken.

The act of sharing your story is undeniably powerful, yet it comes with its own set of challenges and considerations.

The first step is ensuring your emotional readiness.

Sharing may reopen old wounds or expose you to public scrutiny. It's important to assess whether you're emotionally stable enough to handle potential reactions—both positive and negative.

If you decide to share, please start in a supportive environment. This might be a small support group or with a therapist who offers a safe space for those first words.

Your initial sharing attempts will serve as *litmus tests* for how you might feel sharing more publicly, such as in community forums or larger advocacy platforms.

- ✓ **Choosing where and how you share is just as important as deciding when.**

In today's digital age, numerous platforms are available, from social media to blogs to speaking at events.

Each platform has its own audience and mode of interaction. Consider what level of engagement and visibility you are comfortable engaging.

Example: Writing a blog allows for more controlled and thoughtful expression. It's a powerful way to reach others without the immediacy of face-to-face interactions. On the other hand, speaking at events may have an immediate impact but also requires a greater level of public exposure.

No matter the platform you choose, ensure it's one where you feel your voice is respected and protected.

Advocacy: Help Yourself and Others

Believe it or not, you are something of an expert.

- ✓ **For better or worse, you have a unique brand of understanding C-PTSD that cannot be learned in a university.**

You have *lived experiences* and real-time information that needs to be added to the knowledge repository of PTSD management and recovery.

Engaging in advocacy work may further assist your journey and broaden the impact of your story.

Advocating for PTSD awareness not only educates the public. Advocacy also influences policy and supports the development of better resources.

It fosters a more compassionate society that understands and supports the nuances of trauma recovery.

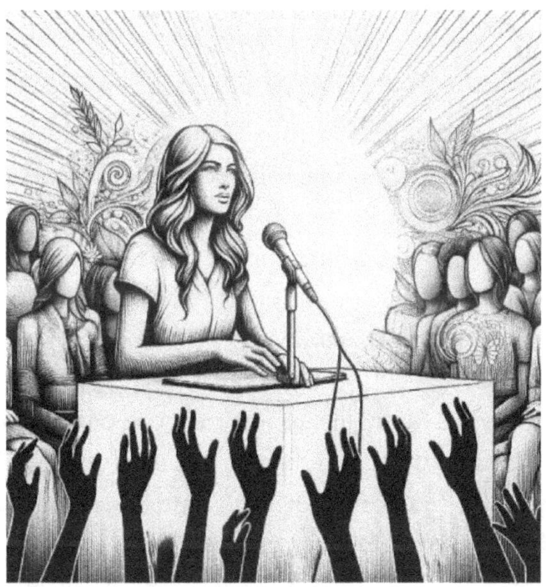

Advocacy can be particularly impactful in military communities, where the culture around mental health is still evolving.

You might choose to collaborate with existing organizations that align with your values.

You may even start your own initiatives that address the gaps you've identified in support and resources.

Advocating for Yourself

- ✓ **You are your most important advocate**.

Your responsibility is first to yourself. Help yourself, and then help others. While the benefits of sharing and advocacy are noteworthy, protecting your emotional well-being is paramount.

Set boundaries around how much you share and know when to step back if the emotional toll becomes too great.

Regular check-ins with yourself or with a mental health professional help navigate the emotional highs and lows that come with public exposure.

The value of developing a support network of individuals who understand and offer emotional support cannot be overstated. This network provides a safe harbor when the waves of public engagement become too much.

In choosing to share your story and engage in advocacy, you are taking powerful steps not only in your healing process. You are also reshaping the narrative around trauma, PTSD, C-PTSD, and recovery.

These actions foster your own sense of personal empowerment, all while contributing to a larger movement towards greater awareness, reduced stigma, and enhanced support for all individuals navigating the complexities of trauma.

As you continue to share and advocate, remember that your story is not just a recounting of past events. Your story is a beacon for others living in the darkness. Your story is a testament to the strength and resilience that defines the human spirit.

Wrapping it Up

Let's take a moment to reflect on the ground we've covered.

- In the beginning, we decided to move forward.
- As we traveled along, we decoded the many facets of C-PTSD and explored holistic recovery strategies.
- We blazed a trail interconnecting our minds, bodies, and spirits to environments supportive of recovery.
- We dipped into somatic therapy, embraced the transformative power of creative therapies, and found serenity in nature's embrace.
- Most importantly, we learned the foundational roles that mindfulness and self-compassion play in our healing process.

Our jaunt through these pages highlights several key takeaways. Let's examine them together once more:

1. The importance of recognizing and validating the existence and impact of C-PTSD.
2. The strength and courage of reaching out and asking for help.
3. The deep healing of integrating our body and mind and the irreplaceable solace found in creativity and the natural world.

4. The value of building a supportive lifestyle that fosters resilience, hope, and community.
5. The acceptance that setbacks are a part of recovery and not a sign of failure.
6. The power of giving back and helping others.

Remember, the path to recovery outlined in this book is deeply personal. Each strategy, each narrative shared, is a suggestion awaiting your touch to adapt it to your unique circumstances and needs.

Healing from complex PTSD is not a linear path—it is a continuous process of learning, growth, and adaptation. Stay curious. Remain open to new healing modalities. Above all, be compassionate with yourself.

I cannot stress enough that recovery is indeed possible. Embrace your journey with patience and self-love. Believe in your ability to live a life that is not just survived but richly lived. To every brave soul who has walked through these pages, your resilience is remarkable.

Deciding to confront the shadows of complex PTSD takes courage, and by engaging with this book, you have shown an incredible commitment to your healing process.

- ✓ **You are not alone on this path**.

Your courage is commendable and inspiring. I hope I have offered you solace and practical guidance. I warmly invite you to share your experiences and feedback on this book.

Moving Forward

As we part ways in this book, know that support for your journey doesn't end here. I stand with you in solidarity.

We share not just the struggles but also the victories.

May this book serve as a beacon, a source of comfort, and a guide as you continue to navigate your path to recovery.

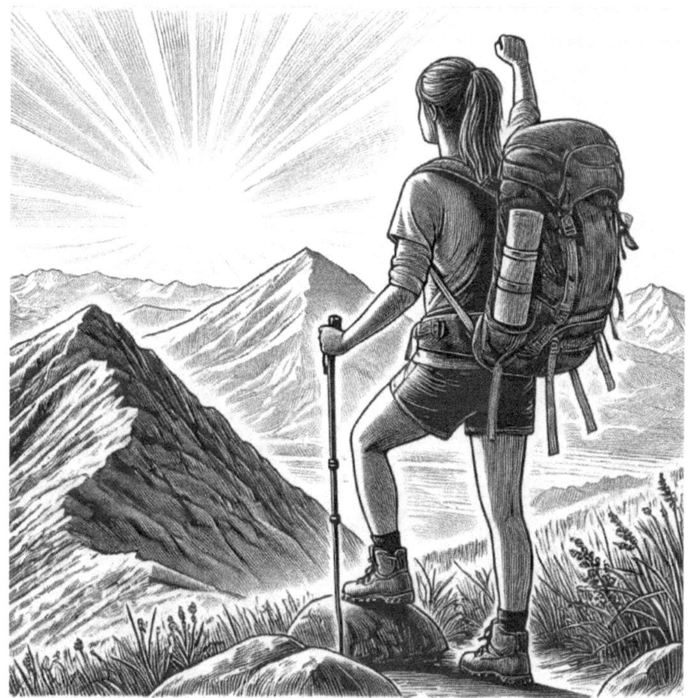

With my deepest respect, Christine Lockhart, PhD.

References

Bagautdinova, D. (2021). The polyvagal theory: New insights into adaptive reactions of the autonomic nervous system. *National Center for Biotechnology Information.* https://www.ncbi.nlm.nih.gov/pmc/articles/PMC3108032/

Cleveland Clinic. (n.d.). CPTSD (Complex PTSD): What it is, symptoms & treatment. *Cleveland Clinic.* https://my.clevelandclinic.org/health/diseases/24881-cptsd-complex-ptsd

Fiore, T. (2023). Grounding techniques to interrupt dissociation. *Psychology Today.* https://www.psychologytoday.com/us/blog/the-discomfort-zone/202302/grounding-techniques-to-interrupt-dissociation

Fiore, T. (2022). How art therapy can heal PTSD. *Healthline.* https://www.healthline.com/health/art-therapy-for-ptsd

First Session. (n.d.). Somatic therapy exercises and techniques. *First Session.* https://www.firstsession.com/resources/somatic-therapy-exercises-techniques

Graham, M. (2022). Healing complex PTSD: Strategies for effective recovery. *Happiness Psychiatrist.* https://www.happinesspsychiatrist.com/post/healing-complex-ptsd

Grow Therapy. (2023). What are SMART therapy goals and why do they matter? *Grow Therapy.* https://growtherapy.com/blog/what-are-smart-goals-in-therapy/

Harvard T.H. Chan School of Public Health. (2021). Associations among PTSD, diet, and gut microbiome. *Harvard T.H. Chan School of Public Health News.* https://www.hsph.harvard.edu/news/press-releases/researchers-discover-associations-among-ptsd-diet-and-the-gut-microbiome/

Huts for Vets. (n.d.). Wilderness therapy program for veterans recovering from trauma. *Huts for Vets.* https://hutsforvets.org/huts-for-vets-wilderness-therapy-program/

Medical News Today. (2023). Complex PTSD and relationships: Effects, triggers, and more. *Medical News Today.* https://www.medicalnewstoday.com/articles/complex-ptsd-triggers-in-relationships

Neel, A. (2022). Therapeutic journaling. *VA.gov Whole Health Library.* https://www.va.gov/WHOLEHEALTHLIBRARY/tools/therapeutic-journaling.asp

Neel, G. (2023). Volunteerism as trauma therapy | Danielle Rousseau. *Boston University Sites.* https://sites.bu.edu/daniellerousseau/2022/04/21/volunteerism-as-trauma-therapy/

Palmer Home for Children. (2022). Designing a healing home: Decorate your space with trauma-informed principles. *Palmer Home.* https://palmerhome.org/designing-a-healing-home-decorate-your-space-with-trauma-informed-principles/

PR Newswire. (2023). New report highlights unique challenges female veterans face after service. *PR Newswire.* https://www.prnewswire.com/news-releases/new-report-highlights-unique-challenges-female-veterans-face-after-service-301931510.html

Sabino Recovery. (2023). How can you rewire your brain after trauma? *Sabino Recovery.* https://www.sabinorecovery.com/rewiring-the-brain-after-trauma/#:~:text=This%20means%20that%20when%20someone,promising%20results%20in%20treating%20PTSD.

WTCFIU. (2023). Finding peace in the night: Sleep hygiene for trauma survivors. *Wellness and Treatment Center at FIU.* https://wtcfl.fiu.edu/finding-peace-in-the-night-sleep-hygiene-for-trauma-survivors/

VA Milwaukee Health Care. (2022). 'This has given me so much': Art therapy keys veteran's recovery. *VA Milwaukee Health Care Stories.* https://www.va.gov/milwaukee-health-care/stories/this-has-given-me-so-much-art-therapy-keys-veterans-recovery/

West Georgia Psychiatric Center. (2022). Ecotherapy: Nature's role in improving mental health. *West Georgia Psychiatric Center.*

https://www.westgeorgiapsychiatriccenter.com/ecotherapy-natures-role-in-improving-mental-health.html

Yoga Journal. (2023). 8 yoga poses to help heal trauma. *Yoga Journal.* https://www.yogajournal.com/practice/yoga-sequences/8-yoga-poses-to-help-heal-trauma/

Zaleski, A. (2023). Routines that help with trauma recovery. *MCCS San Diego.* https://sandiego.usmc-mccs.org/news/routines-that-help-with-trauma-recovery-1#:~:text=Daily%20Routine%20Trauma%20Recovery%20Tips&text=Being%20intentional%20about%20healthy%20daily,you%20get%20through%20the%20day.

Zaleski, A. (2022). Understanding and treating unwanted trauma memories. *National Center for Biotechnology Information.* https://www.ncbi.nlm.nih.gov/pmc/articles/PMC3072671

About the Author

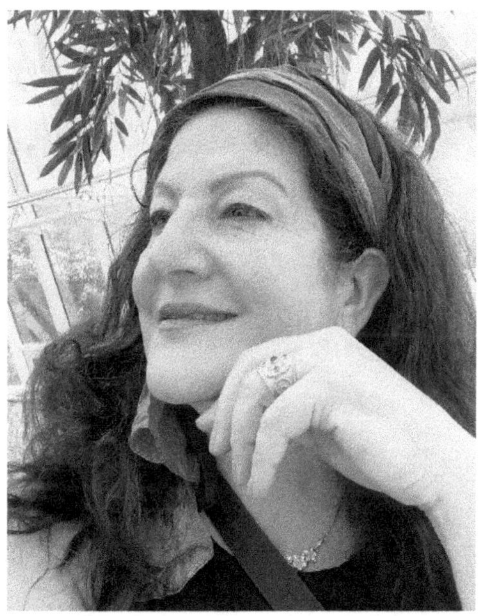

C.W. Lockhart is a trauma survivor. She's also a veteran, a pilgrim, a potter, a writer, and an award-winning professor. Dr. Lockhart has taught writing, literature, art history, management, and organizational leadership in the United States, England, Germany, Ireland, Scotland, Italy, and Japan.

Following 24 years in the Army & Coast Guard, Lockhart embraces the healing modalities of art, nature, pilgrimage, family, and adventure. At home in the world, she claims beautiful coastal Washington as her stateside residence.

Dear Reader,

Thank you so much for reading my book, *Complex PTSD.*

In 10 holistic steps, I've shared real-life tips and strategies that will help you, just as they've helped me.

You have the power to transcend trauma and live your best life.

You can help fellow trauma survivors. How? By reviewing this mighty little book on Amazon.

Please help me spread the good news of recovery. It will just take a second, I promise. And you'll feel good about helping others.

Use the QR code or follow this link:
https://www.amazon.com/review/B0D91H342T

Just a few lines will do. Here are some ideas to get your started:

- What was your favorite part of the book?
- Which strategies did you find the most helpful?
- How has the book made a difference in your life?

Thank you for your trust and support, and for allowing me to be part of your recovery journey. You got this!

Take care & keep shining, Christine Lockhart, PhD

Books by C.W. Lockhart

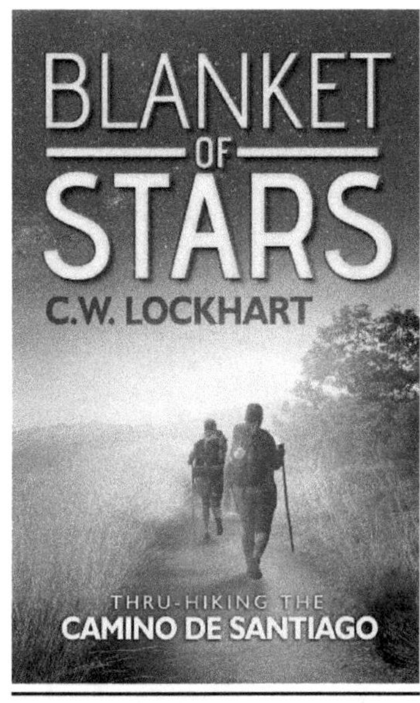

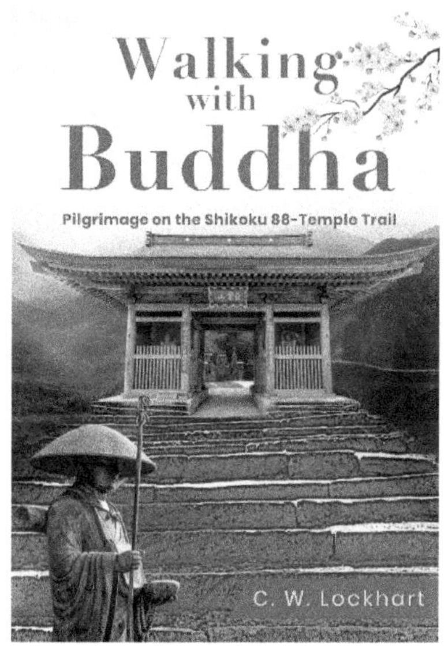

www.ingramcontent.com/pod-product-compliance
Lightning Source LLC
LaVergne TN
LVHW010652110826
845149LV00014B/3050

* 9 7 9 8 9 9 0 9 0 9 1 1 3 *